THE BIGGEST LOSER

BEACH
BODY BLITZ

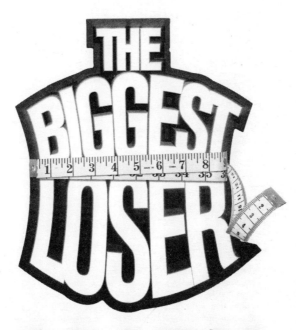

BEACH
BODY BLITZ

Your summer body in
as little as two weeks!

An Hachette UK Company

www.hachette.co.uk

First published in Great Britain in 2011 by Hamlyn,
a division of Octopus Publishing Group Ltd
Endeavour House
189 Shaftesbury Avenue
London WC2H 8JY
www.octopusbooks.co.uk

ISBN 978-0-600-62272-7

A CIP catalogue record for this book is available from the British Library.

Colour reproduction in the UK.

Printed and bound in the UK.

10 9 8 7 6 5 4 3 2 1

General Editor | Gill Paul
Trainer and Consultant | Richard Callender
Recipe Writer | Kate Santon
Senior Editor | Leanne Bryan
Deputy Art Director | Yasia Williams-Leedham
Designer | Jaz Bahra
Copy Editor | Abi Waters
Proofreader | Katie Hardwicke
Indexer | Helen Snaith
Senior Production Controller | Lucy Carter
Publishing Director | Stephanie Jackson

Shine would like to thank: Richard Callender, Wayne Davison, John Gilbert, Jessica
Hannan, Fiona McDonald, Jamie Munro, Claire Nosworthy, Lisa Perrin, Paolo Proto,
Karen Smith, and Gordon Wise of Curtis Brown.

Contents

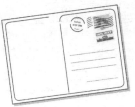

Introduction

Holidays are a time when we should be able to switch off, chill out and forget about our everyday problems and worries. Beach holidays are the most relaxing of all, with warm sun, turquoise sea, golden sand and maybe a gentle breeze rustling the tops of the palm trees. It should be idyllic. But if you are travelling with excess baggage, in the form of a barrel belly, huge, orange-peel thighs and wobbly bingo wings, it could all seem more like a nightmare than a happy dream.

People who are overweight or obese generally do everything in their power to hide their extra rolls of flesh, so the thought of exposing them in swimwear on a public beach is horrifying. There's no place to hide under the sun's glare. You could cower under a giant kaftan but that will only draw attention to your size, making you look like a two-man tent with a head on top. You could make excuses and hide in the hotel room but what's the point in travelling thousands of miles to watch foreign TV? You might as well stay at home with some chocolate and your own remote control.

Holidays are great for our overall health and wellbeing and can leave you feeling refreshed and renewed. Whether you've got 3 or 30 kg (7 or 70 lb) to lose, it would be a shame to miss out because of your body issues and low self-esteem. But some people would do virtually anything to avoid the dreaded swimsuit. They'd rather spend the annual fortnight in bed than on the beach.

WHY HOLIDAYS ARE GOOD FOR YOU

- Your mood is improved and if you have been depressed, a holiday can help to shift it.

- Blood pressure is often lowered on holiday.

- The immune system is boosted, meaning you are less likely to get colds or flu.

- Tense muscles un-knot and hunched shoulders relax.

- You get lots of deep, restful sleep.

- Your mind is rested and you may find that your memory improves as a result.

- Sunlight is one of the best sources of vitamin D available, which helps to protect us from diabetes, osteoporosis and some types of cancer.

- Vitamin D also helps to lower blood cholesterol levels, which could protect us from heart disease.

- Some researchers even think that vitamin D can slow the ageing process.

- The pressures of everyday life, such as commuting and paying bills, are relieved.

- Most people are physically more active on holiday than at home. Not all, but most.

- Heat makes us eat lighter, healthier food than at home.

- You get perspective on your life from a distance and can think clearly about any changes you need to make on your return.

You're reading this book, so you are at least thinking of going on a beach holiday. Maybe some friends or your partner are trying to talk you into it. Perhaps there's an event, such as a wedding, that it would be awkward for you to miss. What we're going to say to you is – just do it! Book that holiday. Do it now. If it's still a few months away, you have time to take your weight in hand and make a real difference, so that you can emerge on the sand feeling confident and happy in your own skin.

On the other hand, it may be that you have already booked the holiday, the departure date is looming and you have only just begun to confront the problem of your jelly belly and thunder thighs. Whatever you do, don't cancel! We can help. You might not be looking like Cheryl Cole or Robert Pattinson by the time your flight is called, but if you start the Beach Body Blitz straight away, we promise you'll look a whole lot better than you do now.

How long have you got?

This plan is designed to last two weeks. We guarantee that you will see dramatic changes if you follow it to the letter, but you have to be strict. No extra slivers of cheese or kids' leftover chicken nuggets can pass your lips during that time. You must do the exercises every morning and evening, no matter what other commitments arise. It's a cumulative process and you won't get the full benefits unless you complete it all.

- If you have two weeks left before your holiday, start now.

- If you have three or four weeks before your holiday, start now and when you finish the two-week plan go back to the beginning and start again.

- If it is more than four weeks until your departure date, follow the advice on pages 209–218 or get hold of the *Biggest Loser: Your Personal Programme for Permanent Weight Loss* and follow that until four weeks before your departure date, at which time, if you still need to, you can use the Beach Body Blitz for a final blast of shaping up.

Why bother?

Maybe you reckon you can put up with the staring eyes on the beach. It's none of their business what you look like, after all. But think about all the other disadvantages of being overweight. You feel the heat much more than your slender mates, and big wet patches form under the armpits of your baggy cotton shirt. It seems as though every part of you sweats, even your hair. You don't have the confidence for shorts

CAUTION

Consult a medical professional before starting this plan if any of the following apply to you:

• You are over forty and need to lose more than a few pounds.

• Your BMI is higher than 29 (see pages 207–208 for information on how to calculate this).

• You haven't exercised for over a year.

• You have been diagnosed with a heart condition, high blood pressure, diabetes, asthma or any other chronic condition that could affect your ability to exercise.

• You have previously experienced chest pains or dizziness that made you lose your balance.

• You have joint or bone problems.

• A doctor has told you to seek advice before starting a diet or an exercise plan.

so tend to cover your legs in long skirts or trousers, raising your core temperature even more. You don't like sleeveless shirts for the same reason, but short-sleeved ones mean you get a tan that stops just above the elbow. You develop a rash in the places where flesh chafes against flesh. Your puffy feet blister in sandals, and your ankles swell up. And all that is without even going into the general health risks of being overweight and unfit.

The bottom line is, don't let your body ruin your holiday. Even with only two weeks to go until your departure date, there's still time to make a difference that could see you stepping onto the sand with renewed confidence, toned and ready to enjoy your well-earned break. And we're sure that once you've seen how easy it is to feel better, you'll want to carry on until you find the perfect body that is buried deep within your present one. This is only the beginning of a whole new you.

CHAPTER ONE

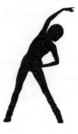

Changing your shape

We can't make you taller or shorter. We can't give you bigger boobs or a broader chest. You're not going to lose 10 kg (22 lb) in two weeks and it would be foolish to try. The bottom line is that if you take a size XXXL, you're not going to be wearing a teensy-weensy bikini – not this year anyway. But if you are prepared to follow every single part of the Beach Body Blitz plan, you will tone, tighten and trim your figure in time for its exposure in swimwear. You will lose some weight as well, but that is not the main point – it's about zapping the blubber and getting some muscle definition showing through.

Fat and firm is infinitely better than fat and wobbly. It doesn't take much to etch the contours of your larger muscles groups, and psychologically this can make a huge difference. A shapely calf, a dimple under the outer shoulder where the deltoid meets the bicep, and the shadow of a quadriceps muscle leading up from the knee – the changes may be subtle but they can affect the way the world perceives you quite dramatically.

*Once you have some muscle definition,
people will see a fit person who might be slightly
overweight rather than a lazy fat person who never
makes an effort. Which would you prefer to be?*

As well as toning your muscles, the Beach Body Blitz is also designed to burn flab, and this can slim your face quite quickly, giving an overall impression of a slimmer person. Once those cheekbones put in an appearance again, that's when friends start asking if you've lost weight – which is always gratifying.

We're not promising miracles – not in two weeks anyway – but we suggest you hold off buying any new clothes for the holiday until a couple of days before departure. There's advice on pages 188–189 about choosing swimwear to flatter your shape, but don't buy holiday dresses, skirts, shorts or t-shirts just yet either. You might find that you'll be able to get into a size that you haven't been close to for years.

CRASH DIETS

You have probably been warned about avoiding crash diets – and those warnings are all correct. If you cut right back on your calorie intake and exist on celery sticks for two weeks, you won't feel very well. You'll put your organs under huge strain, and as soon as you start eating normally again, you will put back on all the weight you have lost – and more. That's because your metabolism thinks it is being starved. It goes into overdrive to protect your vital organs by conserving every last calorie it can as fat to provide stores for the future.

The Beach Body Blitz is different. You will eat nutritious and filling food, with plenty of vitamins and minerals to keep you healthy, while also doing fat-burning and muscle-strengthening exercise. And the more muscle you create, the faster you burn calories, so it's a win-win situation. In Chapter 6 (pages 205–218), you'll find advice on how to make sure you don't put back on any weight you've lost at the end of the plan.

Celebrity bodies

Thank your lucky stars you're not a celebrity, with snappers hiding behind the palm trees ready to immortalize your cellulite or man boobs in the gossip mags. Celebs don't usually control paparazzi shots so can't resort to airbrushing, as they do in pre-arranged magazine shoots, making it much harder to cheat. Of course, some of them have had plastic surgery to get their bodies into shape – boob enhancements, bum lifts and liposuction are all celebrity favourites – but they come at a cost. There's the expense, the risk to health of going under a general anaesthetic, the scars that are left, and the possibility that it could all go wrong and leave you looking worse than when you started. You can often spot the celebs who've had liposuction, for example, as it tends to leave the skin a bit dimply.

We compare ourselves to their on-screen appearances and strive to attain celebrity perfection without thinking about the fact that it took 20 stylists and umpteen hair and make-up people to get them that way. Maybe it's a good thing we can see those paparazzi beach shots and realize that some of them have cellulite, some have more tummy wrinkles than they would like, and many top hunks of the silver screen have a jelly roll above their waistband of their designer shorts. Conversely, certain celebs are way too skinny for their own good. It's only when you see them in beachwear that you realize their ribs protrude like an old-fashioned washboard and they don't have any bottom at all.

Candid celebrity beach shots are useful for reminding us that nobody is perfect. But the ones who do look good on the beach, look good for a reason – because they work at it!

Cameron Diaz, Jennifer Aniston, Elle MacPherson and Helen Mirren (in her 60s!) all look sizzling. So do George Clooney, Jude Law and Zac Efron. And you know why? We are willing to bet our bottom dollar that they all work out virtually every day. Either they have a personal trainer to put them through their paces, or they have the self-discipline to do it themselves. What's more, you are unlikely to see paparazzi shots of them stuffing their faces with cream cakes. They've invested too much hard work in their bodies to fill them with rubbish.

We want you to develop the same attitude: to work hard at slimming and toning your body, then to feel so proud of what you've achieved that you don't jeopardize it by going back to the habits that made you porky in the first place. You don't need a celebrity bank balance when you do it with the Biggest Loser because we'll be your personal trainer, nutritionist and stylist all rolled into one. With us on your side, you too can be a star!

POST-PREGNANCY TUMS

If you've had kids, don't you just hate those celebs who appear on the red carpet six weeks after giving birth looking glowing and perfectly flat-stomached? They've probably got a team of nannies looking after the baby, giving them plenty of time to work out with their trainer and then get a full night's sleep. But they're also likely to be wearing magic knickers and they may have had a quick tummy tuck while they were in hospital. There are even stories of some Hollywood celebs having elective Caesareans at eight months pregnant so they don't get stretched too far out of shape.

Don't compare yourself to them. It can be hard to regain muscle tone post-pregnancy but with perseverance it can be done. Start by focusing on the 'natural girdle' advice on pages 110–113. Do the exercises all day long, whenever you remember, and you'll soon see a difference.

The shape you are in

Our fundamental body shape – width of shoulders and hip bones, length of legs, and the distribution of any fat – is determined by our genes. Girls, if your mother had a small waist and a big butt, chances are you will have as well. Guys, if your dad had a long body and short legs, you may have to learn to live with it.

But the amount of fat and the tone and size of our muscles is in our own hands. These things we can change. If you consume more calories through food than you burn off through exercise, you will lay down extra fat, and if you don't exercise then your muscles will deteriorate. As we get older, our bodies naturally start to lose muscle and we're more prone to laying down fat, but doing enough of the right kind of exercise and watching what we eat can stop the downhill slide.

There's no point in battling against the body shape Mother Nature gave you, but there's plenty you can do to hone and refine that shape, making it the best it can possibly be. There are four basic shapes.

The apple

Do you tend to store excess fat round your middle? Is your waist measurement bigger than your hip measurement? If so, you are in the group that is most at risk of heart disease and diabetes and it's important to take steps to slim down that belly and find the waist that's lurking in there somewhere.

Abdominal fat is bad fat. As well as lying under the skin, it can spread deeper and surround your vital organs, making it hard for them to function efficiently. It causes you to produce an unhealthy kind of blood cholesterol, which can clog up your arteries, and it makes you more prone to several types of cancer. So there are powerful health reasons for getting rid of belly flab, as well as aesthetic reasons. Let's be honest: of all the kinds of fat, it looks worst in swimwear.

Fortunately, there is a lot you can do to trim your mid-section, and you will be able to make a real difference in two weeks if you follow the Beach Body Blitz plan. Find more helpful advice for targeting this area at The Biggest Loser Club (www.biggestloserclub.co.uk).

The pear

Women are more likely to have this body shape than men, and some hate it. Fed up with all the jokes about child-bearing hips and unable to buy dresses because their lower half is two sizes bigger than their chest, they try pounding and pummelling their flesh, targeting it with spot-reduction exercises and frantically rubbing on new 'miracle creams'. But if this is the shape you've inherited, this is the way you will stay.

Narrow shoulders, a flattish chest and wide, curvaceous hips are considered the ideal for women in Latin American countries. Think of all those stunning girls dancing in skimpy bejewelled costumes at the carnival in Rio de Janeiro. They don't think having a big butt is a problem. Over there, it's positively desirable – so long as it is pert and toned. And that's the key. Big, saggy bottoms that overhang lumpy, bumpy thighs are not a thing of beauty. Spend less time sitting on your butt and more time out there getting fit and active, and it will firm up all on its own, without the miracle creams. We'll show you how in the Beach Body Blitz exercise plan on pages 146–153.

The carrot

Broad shoulders and slim hips are the ideal for men in our society, but if you are a skinny carrot rather than a chunky one you might want to focus on developing your chest, arm and shoulder muscles (see pages 154–173).

Women with a carrot shape tend to wish they were a little more curvy. There's not a lot you can do about it, but concentrating on exercises that target the oblique muscles (you'll find some good ones on page 177) can help to create more of a waist.

Carrots should count themselves lucky that of all the body shapes, they are the least likely to lay down fat in the dangerous abdominal area, and the most likely to look good in bikinis or swim shorts.

The hourglass

Big boobs, trim waist and rounded hips is the shape men claim to like best in women, but it takes a lot of work to stay this way. Curvy women are likely to fill out if they're not careful, and can be prone to laying down difficult-to-shift fat in their arms and legs. If they diet, they'll lose weight from their faces or boobs, rather than zapping the thigh wobble and bingo wings. A balanced exercise plan alongside healthy eating is the only way to keep that Marilyn Monroe silhouette, and the younger you are when you start working at it, the more successful you'll be.

After the menopause, hormonal changes can mean that previously hourglass-shaped women start to redistribute the fat that gave them their curves into the mid-section. The look can be more sack of potatoes than sex goddess. But if you establish good muscle tone at a younger age, you'll have a much better chance of staying shapely into old age.

WHAT CAN YOU CHANGE IN TWO WEEKS?

- You can't lose a beer gut that has taken years to reach its current size, but you can reduce it quite significantly. There's probably a lot of bloating under the layers of flab and the Beach Body Blitz plan will target both.

- You can't get rid of lumpy cellulite, but you can tone the underlying muscle and significantly improve the appearance of your thighs and butt, no matter what their size.

- You can't entirely lose a post-pregnancy tummy wobble or make stretch marks vanish, but you can reduce water retention, regain control of your abdominal muscles and rediscover your waist.

- You won't develop Michelle Obama arms if yours currently look like Swiss rolls, but you can tighten those upper arm muscles so there's not quite so much of a swing going on when you wave at someone.

- Getting rid of a double chin takes time, but you will probably slim down your cheeks and bring out those cheekbones.

- And you can make yourself look generally fitter from top to toe.

All that has got to be worth it, don't you think?

STRESS MAKES YOU FAT

It's official! Constantly living life on the edge – wrestling deadlines, dealing with difficult people, battling through heavy traffic, juggling money worries – will trigger the release of a hormone called cortisol that gives us an increased appetite and makes us more likely to lay down excess fat. Stressed people crave high-calorie foods containing sugar and fat as they seek that extra energy burst that will help them solve their current problem. Do you reach for a chocolate hit to help you finish that report on time? Or knock back a few pints of lager after a row with your partner? It may not seem it at the time but you are only making things worse.

In the long term, having high levels of cortisol in your blood makes your body more likely to lay down fat in the abdomen area, and this is when it gets dangerous for health (see page 14). It also raises blood pressure, reduces our resistance to disease and causes our muscles to deteriorate.

You need to find some healthier methods for dealing with stress. And guess what? We have a great suggestion. Exercise is one of the best ways of combating stress, and a regular, ongoing exercise plan will moderate the body's release of stress hormones, making you fitter, healthier and saner too.

Before you start

Those who come to the Biggest Loser boot camp wouldn't dream of letting anyone see them in swimwear. They can't bear to look at themselves unless they're fully clothed (and even then they'd rather not). They avoid having full-length mirrors at home, buy clothes by mail-order and look the other way as they sidle past plate-glass windows to avoid catching a glimpse of their reflection. When it's time for a shower, they strip off and scurry in at top speed without glancing in the bathroom mirror.

The first step is to encourage them to face up to their true condition. And that's what we're going to do with you now. It may seem brutal but it should provide you with the motivation you need to work as hard as you possibly can for the next two weeks of the plan, and to continue making healthy lifestyle choices after the holiday is over. Here's what you have to do:

1 Go to your nearest town centre, taking a camera with you. Walk around until you find a department store that stocks swimwear and has changing rooms with brightly lit, full-length mirrors. If at all possible, find one with mirrors on two walls, so that you can see the back as well as the front view.

2 Select three or four different types of swimwear from the racks, in your current size. Women should choose a couple of bikinis as well as an all-in-one. Men – select some shorter Speedo-style trunks as well as swim shorts.

3 You know what's coming next… try them on and take photos of yourself in the mirror. For each one, take the front view, the side view and, if you can manage, the back view as well.

4 When you get home, take a careful look at the pictures. This is what you are going to look like on the beach unless you pull your finger out and make some changes. That belly is yours and no one else's. Print out the most telling images.

5 Buy a notebook in which to keep your Beach Body Blitz records, and stick the pictures in the front of it. If you wish, you can circle and label the bits you hate the most.

Does the very thought of all this strike fear into your soul? Could you not force yourself to try on swimwear in a department store given the body you're in? Think about it – how on earth are you going to walk out onto a beach then? Do you think it will be easier if you stick your head in the sand?

If it is absolutely impossible for you to get to a department store, and you have a full-length mirror at home, you could delve into the back of a drawer and find a piece of swimwear that used to fit you a few years ago when there was less of you than there is now. Try that on. Look at the way everything bulges over the top and out the sides.

Have a good look. Notice your back fat and your armpit fat as well as the usual belly roll and flabby boobs.

Now take photos. If you have two mirrors, set them up so you can take photos of the back view as well as the front and sides. Apparently, Kate Moss does this in her dressing room at home, so that she knows she can saunter out confidently without some paparazzo catching an unflattering angle.

Stick your photos into a notebook and label them as instructed on the previous page. Now you know the worst, you can start to do something about it. Well done for getting this far! That's the hardest bit out of the way.

Measuring up

Once the ritual humiliation of the 'before' photos is out of the way, it's time to take a full set of measurements. All you'll need is a tape measure. Do this first thing in the morning, either naked or in your underwear. Set out a page in your notebook as follows, and write in all measurements in centimetres (or inches) in the 'before' column.

	BEFORE	AFTER
CHEST (around the nipple line)		
WAIST (the narrowest part)		
MIDRIFF (just over the belly button)		
HIPS (across the tops of the buttocks)		
RIGHT UPPER ARM (the fleshiest bit)		
LEFT UPPER ARM (ditto)		
RIGHT THIGH (the fattest bit)		
LEFT THIGH (ditto)		

The Beach Body Blitz plan is not just about shedding weight, although you will almost certainly do so. The goal of the plan is to trim and tone so you look better on the beach, and your measurements, along with some before and after photos, are going to be the best indicators of success. There's no point in setting weight-loss targets for the two-week period because everyone loses at a different rate. The fatter you are to start off with, the more you are likely to lose. Having said that, seeing the numbers drop can be gratifying, so do step on the scales at the beginning and end of the two-week period. If your scales give body fat percentage, note that at the same time.

	BEFORE	AFTER
WEIGHT (in kg or lb)		
BODY FAT PERCENTAGE		

Moral support

Can you persuade the friends or family members you will holiday with to join you in your Beach Body Blitz? Do any of them need to tone up and trim down? At Biggest Loser we find that having a family member on side is one of the keys to success. They can support you through the tricky moments when motivation is slipping, and celebrate the highs when you start to see results.

It has to be someone who really loves you and doesn't feel remotely competitive with you, though. Beware of the mates who might try to sabotage you, tempting you to come to the pub for a 'quick glass of chilled white' or bringing you a little bar of chocolate as a treat 'because you're doing so well'. Partners can be the worst for this. It's almost as though they don't want you to slim down because they're worried you'll be more attractive to the opposite sex and might be tempted to look elsewhere.

> *If you're going on holiday with friends, there's a chance they'll try to derail your Beach Body Blitz efforts, worried that you will look better than them on a sun lounger.*

Don't be upset about this. It doesn't mean they don't love you. Just let it spur you on and make you even more determined to get in the best possible shape.

See if there is someone reliable who is prepared to do the plan with you. They can partner you at tennis, come for morning runs or swims, and you can cook dinner for each other some evenings. If your willpower weakens at any point, they can direct you back to those 'before' photos and remind you of all the reasons why it's important for you to shape up – and you can do the same for them.

What you will need

On pages 28–29, you'll find a shopping list of foods you'll have to stock up on to follow the eating plan. Buy these the day before you are planning to start (or straight away if your departure date is imminent). At the same time, it's a good idea to clear your cupboards of any junk food that could undermine your resolve. You know what your own particular weaknesses are. Is it sweets, crisps, cake, biccies, cheese, bread or ice cream that tends to be your downfall? Ignore the protests of your family and load these into a box for disposal. Give them to a skinny friend, or take them to a shelter for the homeless if you can't face chucking them in the bin.

Every morning for the duration of the plan, you will be doing 45 minutes of aerobic exercises. Read the suggestions on pages 119–135 and decide which ones you want to do. Choose at least two different kinds, preferably more, so you don't get bored. Then check what you will need to do them.

- Buy the correct kind of shoes for your chosen exercise.
- You'll find stockists of hula hoops, skipping ropes, rollerblades and trampolines listed on page 223.
- Do you want to join a local gym to do your aerobic exercise? Better get that application in.
- Is there a swimming pool you can use nearby?
- Where can you go canoeing or play ball sports nearby?
- Any good dance classes locally?
- If you want to work out to exercise DVDs or Wii Fit, now's the time to buy them. Why not try one of the Biggest Loser workout DVDs?
- You'll wear light, comfortable clothing in layers, and a water bottle will come in handy.

The second part of the exercise plan is a toning regime called 'The Resistance Workout' (see pages 136–185). To do this, you'll need just a few items:

- A pair of dumbbells – as heavy as you can manage without straining. Women can usually manage between 4–8 kg (8–17 lb), and men between 6–12 kg (13–26 lb).
- A resistance band. These are usually sold in three strengths: for beginners, intermediate and advanced. Choose the right one for your level.
- An exercise mat or rug, some cushions and a rolled-up towel. You'll find stockists of weights and other exercise equipment on page 223.

Ready? Get set… Go…

If there are fewer than four weeks to go before your departure date, start the plan straight away. Once you get to the end of the two-week plan, you can go back and start it again, continuing right up till the day you leave. If there are more than four weeks to go, turn to pages 209–218 for advice on making lifestyle changes to lose weight permanently. Alternatively, log on to The Biggest Loser Club (www.biggestloserclub.co.uk) to check out all sorts of helpful tips, advice, recipes and exercises to continue your progress.

Don't do the Beach Body Blitz plan for any more than four weeks. It's not designed as a long-term eating and exercise plan.

This is a quick-fix plan with the main aim of making you look better in swimwear. We're appealing shamelessly to your vanity! Sure, it will make you healthier as well, but psychologically it wouldn't work for longer than four weeks. Apart from anything else, you'd never keep up those two obligatory exercise sessions a day. Come on, you know you wouldn't!

CHART YOUR PROGRESS

Keeping a note of how you're doing is good for morale, building a sense of achievement as the days go by. Assign a page in your notebook for each day of the Beach Body Blitz plan, and write Day 1, Day 2... at the top. You will find the menu plans for each day on pages 31–37 and we advise that you stick to these exactly, but if for any reason you have to vary them (maybe swapping lunches with another day because you've run out of a key ingredient) then you should note this down. If you slip up and eat something that's not on the plan, note that down too. Otherwise, just write Breakfast, Lunch, Dinner, Snack, and give yourself a big tick next to each of them.

Below this, write down the aerobic exercise you completed each day and how long you did it for, then note the number of repetitions you managed in the Resistance Workout. We want you to set yourself challenges in both exercise sessions and try to achieve more each day. This will keep it interesting, as well as increasing your calorie burn and muscle build. And at the end, you can look back and feel proud.

As you start, keep thinking of all the benefits you will see – even if you're only doing it for two weeks.

- You will have more defined muscles.
- You will get rid of any bloating, water retention and a fair bit of flab.
- You will feel healthy and full of energy.
- Your skin will be clearer and your eyes sparkling.
- Your digestive system will be working more efficiently.
- Your posture will improve.
- And finally – all-important as you prepare to expose it in swimwear – your flesh won't wobble so much!

CHAPTER TWO

The eating plan

There are dozens of diets out there that could help you to lose a bit of weight in time for your holiday, even if you only have two weeks to go. However, most of them tend to severely restrict the number and quantity of foods you can eat, so that you spend your time starving, bored and lacking in energy.

The very low-calorie plans can't be combined with an exercise plan because you would simply collapse with fatigue. The absolutely-no-carbs-at-all plans make you constipated, give you bad breath and can put a strain on your heart and vital organs. And many other plans are simply too fiddly to follow.

The Beach Body Blitz eating plan is different from all of these. You will be able to eat lots of fruits and vegetables, fish and chicken, delicious soups and salads that can be prepared in advance for a working lunch, mouth-watering smoothies, low-cal snacks and tasty, easy-to-cook dinners that are filling enough to serve to all the family. There will be plenty of fibre to get your digestive system moving, plus enough food that you should never be hungry, whilst containing fewer calories than you're used to, so you will start dropping kilos (pounds). And it's really easy to follow!

*Each day you will be given a menu plan that has
been carefully designed to contain 1,500 kcal
for women and 1,750 kcal for men.*

These calorie limits are low enough that you will definitely lose weight. Combining them with the exercise plan will mean you lose more weight, but you won't make yourself ill. Don't try to eat any less than these limits, say by skipping a meal or reducing the quantities, or you risk bringing on the 'crash diet effect' when your body goes into starvation mode and stores calories as fat. Follow the plan exactly and you'll reap the benefits.

Here are a few general rules you should know before you start:

- You can switch meals around to an extent within the 14-day plan, for example having Day 3's lunch on Day 2, but aim to eat all the meals during the 14 days to ensure you get a balanced range of nutrients.

- Don't switch lunches and dinners. This is because lunches contain carbohydrates and you won't be eating any carbs in the evenings (see page 26).

- It's fine if you don't feel like eating breakfast until mid-morning, although if you work away from home you will need to choose a breakfast option that can be transported, such as the Swiss muesli or date and fruit yogurt (see page 31).

- Try not to have dinner too late or you won't have time to digest it properly before you go to bed.

- Don't eat out during the plan, unless you are invited to dinner with a friend who is also following it and will cook the appropriate meal for you. You have no control over portion sizes in restaurants, and you don't know what hidden fats they may have added.

- All your ingredients should be fresh or frozen and cooked from scratch. Don't use pre-prepared meals from supermarkets or ready-cook sauces from a jar.

- Measure your portion sizes carefully. Remember: excess portions contain excess calories.

- You don't need to count calories on the Beach Body Blitz eating plan, because we've done it all for you, but don't forget about calories altogether. For example, be aware that an extra knob of butter on your bread can add 50 kcal, and a tablespoon of olive oil has 135 kcal. Little extras soon add up.

Covering all the food groups

Our bodies need nutrients from a wide range of different foods to remain healthy, and some of them are especially important when you are following an exercise plan. Unlike some other weight-loss plans, we would never recommend cutting an entire food group. Beach Body Blitz is a balanced diet including all the nutrients you need.

Protein
This is essential for building muscle and helping you to burn calories. It stops you feeling hungry between meals, and makes you more alert and less tired. You'll get plenty of high-quality protein from the fish, chicken, eggs, cheese and pulses in our eating plan.

Carbs
When you eat starchy carbs, such as bread, pasta, rice and potatoes, your digestive system breaks them down into glucose (a type of sugar), which is either stored in your muscles to supply energy for activity, or in the fat cells, where it creates extra blubber. If you eat them in the evening when your system is slowing down, the latter is more likely and that's why you shouldn't eat any starchy carbs after 6pm on this plan. There are plenty to eat earlier in the day, with sufficient fibre to keep things moving smoothly through your digestive system, and enough B vitamins for good health.

Fats
Fats are necessary for cooking food and making it palatable, and they also help to make you feel fuller, so it's a mistake to cut them entirely. But there are good fats and bad fats (see page 101), and we're focusing on the good ones on this plan – in moderation.

Vitamins and minerals
You will easily get your five a day on the eating plan, and you'll be eating lots of different types of fruit and veg at every meal. There is a certain amount of licence to make substitutions if, for example, you really can't stand broccoli – but don't limit your selection to just carrots or only apples. Lots of different coloured fruits and veggies are necessary to provide all the nutrients your body needs.

Portion sizes calculator

It's recommended that you weigh portions carefully, using scales or measuring jugs and spoons. Slimmers' scales are widely available and useful for measuring small quantities that can make a big difference in calorie terms. Here is a quick calculator for when you are in a hurry:

• 30 g (1 oz) wholegrain porridge oats is about 3 level tablespoons.
• 25 g (1 oz) brown rice (uncooked) is about 1.25 tablespoons.
• 50 g (2 oz) Puy lentils (uncooked) is about 4 tablespoons.
• 100 g (3½ oz) feta cheese is half a standard block.
• A slim round of goats' cheese weighs about 80 g (3 oz).
• A small carton of yogurt is 150 g (5 oz).
• A 150 g (5 oz) chicken breast is medium and 250 g (8 oz) is large.
• An average fillet of salmon would be about 150 g (5 oz).
• 100 g (3½ oz) of berries or chopped fruit would fill half a cup.
• 10 g (½ oz) dried fruit is about 1 tablespoon.

Do double check whenever you have the time because the calorie differences can be really substantial, especially with nuts, oils and dairy products.

WATER

It's important that you stay hydrated on the Beach Body Blitz plan, so get into the habit of having a glass of water beside you at work or at home, and carrying a little bottle with you whenever you are outdoors or exercising. Water helps your digestive system to absorb vital nutrients and then flush waste products through your system. It makes you feel fuller, as well. Often when you think you feel hungry, you are actually mildly dehydrated and a big glass of water will do the trick. For other drinks you can have on the Beach Body Blitz plan, see pages 104–105.

Your Beach Body Blitz shopping list

Fruit and vegetables
Apples (inc. dessert apples)
Oranges (inc. satsumas, clementines)
Kiwifruit
Grapes (green, red and black)
Strawberries
Blueberries
Peaches
Watermelon
Galia melon
Bananas
Lemons
Red plums
Any other favourite fruits

Aubergine
Mushrooms (button and large flat ones)
Spinach
French beans
Broccoli
Mangetout
Pak choi
Red and yellow peppers
Red and white onions
Garlic
Carrots
New potatoes
Courgettes
Beetroot
White cabbage
Fennel
Celery
Celeriac root
Any other favourite vegetables

Salad leaves (including watercress and rocket)

Cucumber
Spring onions and shallots
Tomatoes (large and cherry)

Fresh basil
Fresh chives
Fresh coriander
Fresh parsley
Fresh thyme
Fresh mint
Fresh root ginger
Red chillies (optional)

Protein
Eggs
Sardines in oil (canned)
Tuna in spring water (canned)
Fresh tuna steak
Cooked and raw king prawns
Salmon fillet
Cod loin, or other white fish
Smoked haddock
Smoked mackerel
Chicken breasts

Dairy
Feta cheese
Goats' cheeses of your choice (see page 73)
Greek 0%-fat yogurt
Natural low-fat yogurt
Low-fat mayonnaise

Carbs
Wholegrain porridge oats
Wheat-free bread and brown rolls (see box opposite)
Oatcakes
Brown rice

Chickpeas (tinned)
Puy lentils (dried)

Fats
Olive oil
Vegetable oil spray
Sesame oil
Olive-oil spread
Unsalted butter

Storecupboard essentials
Dried apricots
Dried cranberries or blueberries
Prunes
Dried figs
Raisins
Sultanas
Dates

Sesame seeds
Pumpkin seeds
Almonds
Cashew nuts
Walnuts
Pine nuts
Any other favourite nuts

Herbs and spices (including cinnamon, bay leaves, paprika, garam masala, cumin, lemon grass, cayenne pepper, mixed herbs, ground ginger)
Mustard seeds
Dijon and wholegrain mustard
Balsamic vinegar
Tabasco sauce
Soy sauce
Chicken stock (cubes or jarred)
Marmite (optional)

Tomato passata
Tomato purée
Tahini paste
Capers (optional)
Black and green olives
Anchovy fillets (optional)

Earl Grey tea bags
Green and white tea
Herbal teas of all kinds (chamomile, peppermint, nettle, fennel, fruits, or any other favourites)

WHEAT-FREE BREAD

Most supermarkets and health food stores offer a range of wheat-free breads, but if yours doesn't you can order some on the internet (see page 223 for stockists). Choose from brown rice bread, rye, pumpernickel, amaranth, quinoa, flax, buckwheat, corn, chestnut, linseed, millet, spelt, oat and hemp breads, with or without seeds, such as pumpkin, sesame, lupin and sunflower. Read the packaging and try to find a loaf in which a slice of bread comes in at 75 kcal. You will also need some small brown rolls with about 150 kcal each.

The menu plans

It will be simplest if you stick to the menu plans for the 14 days exactly as they are laid out on pages 31–37. However, if you haven't managed to buy any fish on a day when it's on the menu for dinner you can swap with another dinner menu that has a similar calorie count. Or perhaps you have to be out of the house and can't make yourself a hot lunch, in which case you can swap with a lunch that can be easily transported in a lunchbox. Or swap whole days if that's easiest, for example having the Day 13 menu on Day 10 and vice versa.

Try to have each lunch and dinner once in the 14 days to get all the nutrients you need for good health. And don't swap lunches with dinners and vice versa.

There are only five different breakfasts listed, because most of us are creatures of habit at breakfast-time. If you love the muesli or the date and fruit yogurt, you can have them any day you like. You may want to save cooked breakfasts for weekends when you have more time – but be aware that protein breakfasts (with eggs or fish) will make you feel full for longer so are a good idea if you're not going to be able to have a mid-morning snack.

Try to vary the snacks you choose instead of opting for the same ones every time. Eat them at the time of day when you get peckish, whether that's mid-morning, mid-afternoon or in the evening, but remember not to eat snacks with carbs (such as oatcakes or bread) after 5pm.

Ready to begin?
Here are the menus.

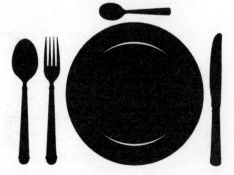

Day 1

Breakfast
Swiss muesli with orange and apple (see page 39).

Lunch
Gazpacho, served with oatcakes and sardines (see page 45).

Dinner
Chicken and pepper casserole (see page 61).
Your choice of the fruit salads (see pages 82–83).

Snacks
Women can choose a 100-calorie snack (see pages 87–88)
and a 50-calorie snack (see page 86).
Men can choose one substantial snack (see pages 88–91)
and two 100-calorie snacks (see pages 87–88).

–

Day 2

Breakfast
Date and fruit yogurt with almonds (see page 41).

Lunch
Chickpea salad with tuna, red onion and garlic croûtons
(see page 52).

Dinner
Omelette with soft goats' cheese and a tomato salad (see page 62).
Pan-fried apples with cinnamon (see page 81).

Snacks
Women can choose two 50-calorie snacks (see page 86).
Men can choose one substantial snack (see pages 88–91),
one 100-calorie snack (see pages 87–88)
and one 50-calorie snack (see page 86).

Day 3

Breakfast
Poached egg and spinach, with two slices of toast (see page 40).

Lunch
Tangy hummous with crudités (see page 48).

Dinner
Grilled tuna steak with rocket and green salad (see page 63).
Plum compôte with toasted almonds (see page 80).

Snacks
Women can choose two 100-calorie snacks (see pages 87–88).
Men can choose two substantial snacks (see pages 88–91),
or four 100-calorie snacks (see pages 87–88).

–

Day 4

Breakfast
Lemony smoked haddock, with two slices of toast (see page 42).

Lunch
Roasted beetroot and feta salad (see page 50).

Dinner
Aubergine curry with green beans and cucumber raita (see page 64).
Warm grilled peaches with pine nuts or almonds (see page 84).

Snacks
Women can choose one substantial snack (see pages 88–91)
and one 100-calorie snack (see pages 87–88).
Men can choose two substantial snacks (see pages 88–91)
and one 50-calorie snack (see page 86).

Day 5

Breakfast
Swiss muesli with orange and apple (see page 39).

Lunch
North Indian carrot salad with cashew nuts in a baked potato
(see page 49).

Dinner
Aromatic salmon in a parcel, served with steamed pak choi, mangetout,
broccoli or green salad with lemon dressing (see page 66).
Your choice of the fruit salads (see pages 82–83).

Snacks
Women can choose two 100-calorie snacks (see pages 87–88).
Men can choose two substantial snacks (see pages 88–91),
or four 100-calorie snacks (see pages 87–88).

–

Day 6

Breakfast
Scrambled egg with mushrooms and two slices of toast (see page 44).

Lunch
Carrot and orange soup, with a brown roll and feta cheese
(see page 46).

Dinner
Roast chicken pieces with lemon and herbs, served with salad
(see page 67).
Apple compôte with yogurt (see page 80).

Snacks
Women can choose two 100-calorie snacks (see pages 87–88).
Men can choose two substantial snacks (see pages 88–91),
or four 100-calorie snacks (see pages 87–88).

Day 7

Breakfast
Poached egg and spinach, with two slices of toast (see page 40).

Lunch
Prawn and melon salad with a wheat-free roll (see page 57).

Dinner
Stuffed pepper and courgette with a yogurt sauce (see page 68).
Dried fruit salad (see page 85).

Snacks
Women can choose a 100-calorie snack (see pages 87–88)
and a 50-calorie snack (see page 86).
Men can choose one substantial snack (see pages 88–91)
and two 100-calorie snacks (see pages 87–88).

–

Day 8

Breakfast
Swiss muesli with orange and apple (see page 39).

Lunch
Crunchy coleslaw, with a wheat-free brown roll (see page 53).

Dinner
Chicken stir-fry with oriental vegetables and cashew nuts
(see page 70).
Your choice of the fruit salads (see pages 82–83).

Snacks
Women can choose two 50-calorie snacks (see page 86).
Men can choose one substantial snack (see pages 88–91)
and one 100-calorie snack (see pages 87–88).

Day 9

Breakfast
Date and fruit yogurt with almonds (see page 41).

Lunch
New potato salad with cherry tomatoes, herbs and smoked mackerel
(see page 51).

Dinner
Roasted vegetables with grilled goats' cheese (see page 72).
Your choice of the fruit salads (see pages 82–83).

Snacks
Women can choose one 50-calorie snack (see page 86).
Men can choose three 100-calorie snacks (see pages 87–88).

–

Day 10

Breakfast
Scrambled egg with mushrooms and two slices of toast (see page 44).

Lunch
Lentil, tomato and goats' cheese salad (see page 55).

Dinner
Prawns in garlicky tomato sauce (see page 71).
Plum compôte with toasted almonds (see page 80).

Snacks
Women can choose one 100-calorie snack (see pages 87–88)
and one 50-calorie snack (see page 86).
Men can choose two substantial snacks (see pages 88–91)
or four 100-calorie snacks (see pages 87–88).

Day 11

Breakfast
Swiss muesli with orange and apple (see page 39).

Lunch
Minestrone, with 3 black pepper oatcakes and goats' cheese
(see page 47).

Dinner
Salade Niçoise (see page 76).
Pan-fried apples with cinnamon (see page 81).

Snacks
Women can choose two 50-calorie snacks (see page 86).
Men can choose one substantial snack (see pages 88–91)
and one 100-calorie snack (see pages 87–88).

–

Day 12

Breakfast
Date and fruit yogurt with almonds (see page 41).

Lunch
Feta dip with crudités (see page 54).

Dinner
Fish plaki, served with steamed broccoli, mangetout or a green salad
with lemon dressing (see page 74).
Warm grilled peaches with pine nuts or almonds (see page 84).

Snacks
Women can choose two 50-calorie snacks (see page 86).
Men can choose one substantial snack (see pages 88–91)
and one 100-calorie snack (see pages 87–88).

Day 13

Breakfast
Lemony smoked haddock, with two slices of toast (see page 42).

Lunch
Hot chicken-strip salad (see page 58).

Dinner
Grilled mushrooms with spinach and cheese (see page 77).
Dried fruit salad (see page 85).

Snacks
Women can choose two 100-calorie snacks (see pages 87–88)
and one 50-calorie snack (see page 86).
Men can choose two substantial snacks (see pages 88–91)
and one 50-calorie snack (see page 86).

–

Day 14

Breakfast
Poached egg and spinach, with two slices of toast (see page 40).

Lunch
Celeriac remoulade with a baked potato (see page 56).

Dinner
Pan-fried crispy salmon with courgettes and lemon mayonnaise
(see page 78).
Your choice of the fruit salads (see pages 82–83).

Snacks
Women can choose two 100-calorie snacks (see pages 87–8).
Men can choose one substantial snack (see pages 88–91)
and two 100-calorie snacks (see pages 87–8).

Beach Body Blitz recipes

None of these recipes are difficult to make, even if you are not used to wielding a spatula. In fact, it doesn't matter if you've never cooked in your life before. You will manage these dishes because we've explained all the basics such as how to poach an egg or bake a potato. You don't need any more complex kitchen equipment than some measuring scales, a blender and a few pots and pans. A lot of dishes just require some chopping and mixing then gentle heating.

Most recipes give a single serving, but in some cases it is more practical to make a larger quantity – enough for two. Freeze the second portion (if no-one else wants it) and you'll have your very own ready meals.

Remember to weigh and measure ingredients carefully. Slimmers' scales are a good investment for weighing smaller quantities accurately. All spoon measurements are for level spoonfuls, unless stated otherwise. Weights for plain salad leaves are not given – you can eat a lot of salad leaves without adding many calories, unless you cover them in dressing, so have as much as you want.

Remember that all bread and rolls are wheat-free varieties. The bread should have 75 kcal per slice and a brown roll should have 150 kcal.

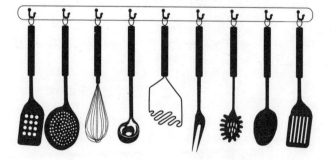

BREAKFASTS
Calories 400 kcals | **Serves** 1

Swiss muesli with orange and apple

This muesli is simply delicious, and easy to make. We think you'll love it. If you don't have time to cook in the morning, you can substitute this for any other breakfast.

30 g (1 oz) wholegrain porridge oats
4 large ready-to-eat dried apricots
1 date
5 whole almonds
4 hazelnuts
1 teaspoon pumpkin seeds
1 teaspoon sunflower seeds
Juice of half a large orange
1 apple

1 Prepare the muesli base the evening before. Put the oats into a bowl, then chop the apricots, date, almonds and hazelnuts and add them. Scatter in the pumpkin and sunflower seeds and mix everything together. Add the orange juice and stir well. Cover the bowl with clingfilm and leave it in the fridge overnight.

2 The following morning, core and chop the apple finely – leave the peel on – and stir it into the muesli. Serve immediately.

TIP
Find more great breakfast recipes like this at The Biggest Loser Club (www.biggestloserclub.co.uk).

Calories 350 kcals (including the toast) I **Serves** 1

Poached egg and spinach with toast

If your poached eggs normally distintegrate, try our method
– or buy an egg poacher for perfect results every time.
Remember: protein breakfasts will make you feel fuller for
longer so are great for busy mornings.

150–200 g (5–7 oz) baby spinach leaves
1 large egg
1 ¼ teaspoons vegetable or olive oil
Salt and black pepper

To serve:
2 slices of wheat-free bread, toasted, with olive-oil spread

1   Wash the spinach and squeeze any excess moisture out, then chop
    the leaves. It will look like a huge amount, but will cook down.

2   Set a pan of water on to boil, and crack the egg into a small bowl.
    If you are using an egg poacher, add a drop of oil to the poaching
    cup. Reduce the water to a simmer and add the poaching cup, then
    slide the egg into it. Alternatively, poach it directly in the water –
    just swirl the simmering water and then tip the egg into the middle.
    Cook until the egg white is set – about 4 minutes or so.

3   While the egg is cooking, put the spinach into a large pan over a
    medium heat. Add some black pepper and a small pinch of salt and
    cook until it is soft; this happens quite quickly and does not require
    any additional liquid. Drain the spinach and put it on a warmed
    plate – squeeze any more excess liquid out if necessary.

4   Put the poached egg on top and serve immediately, accompanied
    by the toast.

BREAKFASTS
Calories 390 kcals | **Serves** 1

Date and fruit yogurt with almonds

A creamy, crunchy, sweet treat to waken your taste buds.
If you haven't had time to breakfast at home, you can prepare
this with untoasted almonds while you are out and about.

150 g (5 oz) Greek 0%-fat yogurt
1 dessert apple or half a large banana
6 dates
7 whole almonds

1 Empty the yogurt into a serving bowl. Chop the apple, or peel and
chop the banana, and add it to the yogurt. Stir it in well, then chop
the dates and add them too; stir again.

2 Put a small frying pan on a high heat and roughly chop the almonds
while it is heating up. When the pan is hot, tip the almonds in and
toast them, stirring constantly until they start to brown. Then take
the pan off the heat and scatter the toasted almonds over the
yogurt; serve immediately.

TIP
Try The Biggest Loser meal replacement range for snack bars that
make a great alternative to these breakfasts for days when you're
busy and on the go all morning.

Lemony smoked haddock with toast

Just 2 minutes in the microwave or 5 minutes on the hob
(see box opposite), and you'll have a high-protein, low-fat
breakfast fit for beachwear models.

1 piece of undyed smoked haddock, about 200 g (7 oz)
Juice of half a large lemon
A little parsley
¼ teaspoon Dijon mustard

To serve:
2 slices of wheat-free bread, toasted, with olive-oil spread

1 The easiest – and least smelly – way to cook this is in the
microwave. Put the piece of haddock in a microwaveable dish, then
add 1 teaspoon of lemon juice and 2 tablespoons of water. Cover
the dish with clingfilm, pierce the film in two or three places and
microwave for about 2 minutes at 800 watts (adjust the time for
different wattage ovens) until cooked; it is done when the flesh is
opaque and flakes easily. Chop the parsley and set it to one side.

2 While the fish is cooking, put the rest of the lemon juice in a small
pan, add the mustard and stir well. Warm it over a medium heat.
When the fish is ready, remove the clingfilm and drain the juices
into the pan, then cover the dish with the haddock in it to keep
the fish warm. Bring the lemony liquid to the boil and boil it rapidly
until the liquid has reduced by about half. Put the fish on a plate
and pour the sauce over it, then scatter with the parsley – and
serve immediately with 2 slices of wheat-free toast.

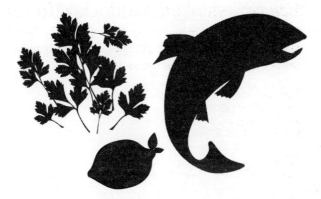

ON THE HOB

If you don't have a microwave, you can cook your fish on the hob. Put enough water in a shallow pan to just cover the fish, and bring it to a gentle simmer. When it reaches simmering point, add 1 teaspoon lemon juice and then slide the fish in. Cover the pan and poach the haddock for about 5 minutes, depending on the thickness of the fish. Lift it out of the pan when it is cooked (the flesh will be opaque) and keep it warm. Use 2 tablespoons of the poaching liquid to make the sauce with the rest of the lemon juice and mustard, as described in the main recipe.

Scrambled egg with mushrooms and toast

Don't overcook the eggs or they'll be rubbery instead of creamy. Adventurous souls could use different types of mushrooms with stronger flavours.

2 eggs
150 g (5 oz) button mushrooms
1 teaspoon olive-oil spread
Black pepper

To serve:
2 slices of wheat-free bread, toasted, with olive-oil spread

1 Beat the eggs in a bowl and add a little black pepper to season. Then prepare the mushrooms: wipe them clean and cut in half. Warm half of the olive-oil spread in a small nonstick frying pan and add the mushrooms. Cook them for a couple of minutes and then increase the heat.

2 Put the rest of the spread in a nonstick saucepan over a medium heat and allow it to melt. Give the egg another quick beat, then pour it into the pan. Leave it for a minute then stir with a wooden spoon. Keep an eye on the mushrooms at the same time; if they are giving off a lot of liquid, increase the heat and let it cook off. Just before the eggs look set, take the saucepan off the heat; they will finish cooking in the heat of the pan.

3 Put the cooked mushrooms on a plate, add the scrambled egg and serve immediately, accompanied with 2 slices of wheat-free toast.

Gazpacho

The fabulous summery flavours of Spain's famous cold soup will give you a taste of your beach holiday before you leave home.

1 red pepper
Half a cucumber
1 small red onion
150 g (5 oz) ripe tomatoes
1 garlic clove, crushed
500 ml (17 fl oz) tomato passata
1 teaspoon balsamic vinegar
Salt and black pepper
Ice cubes

To serve, per person:
60 g (2¼ oz) tinned sardines in oil
2 plain oatcakes

1 Cut the pepper in half and discard the white membrane and seeds, then chop one half and set it to one side. Chop half of the cucumber and onion, then chop most of the tomatoes (reserving 1 to keep whole), and remove as many of the seeds as possible.

2 Put the garlic in a blender. Add the passata and the chopped pepper, cucumber, onion and tomatoes (put the unchopped vegetables into a container, cover and refrigerate). Add the vinegar and blend the soup well, then push it through a sieve into a bowl. Add a little cold water if the purée seems too thick, but it is not supposed to be watery. Cover the bowl and chill the soup in the fridge for at least 1 hour.

3 Before serving, dice the remaining pepper, cucumber, onion and tomato finely. Drain the sardines, pat them dry, then crush them lightly onto 2 oatcakes. To serve the gazpacho, put a couple of ice cubes in a bowl and spoon the soup over them. Sprinkle the chopped vegetables over the bowl of gazpacho, and accompany with the oatcakes and sardines.

LUNCHES
Calories 395 kcals | **Serves** 2

30 kcal more if you use olive-oil spread on the roll but try it first –
you shouldn't need it.

Carrot and orange soup

Carrot and orange are a match made in heaven. This is so
delicious you could serve it at a gourmet dinner party and
have everyone begging for the recipe.

1 teaspoon vegetable oil
1 onion, chopped
1 garlic clove, finely chopped
1 orange
400 g (13 oz) carrots, chopped
1 potato, peeled and chopped
Salt and black pepper

To serve, per person:
1 small wheat-free brown roll
25 g (1 oz) feta cheese

1 Warm the oil in a large pan over a medium heat, add the chopped
   onion and garlic and cook gently for 5 minutes, until it begins to
   soften. While the onion is cooking, squeeze the orange juice into
   a small bowl. Once the onion is soft, add the carrots and potato
   to the pan and stir well, then add the orange juice.

2 Add enough water to the pan to cover the vegetables and increase
   the heat. Bring the soup to the boil, then reduce the heat and
   simmer, covered, until the vegetables are soft – about 10 minutes.

3 Liquidize the soup, and if it seems thick, add a little more water
   and blend again to get the consistency you prefer. Reheat the
   soup, check the seasoning and serve, accompanied with a wheat-
   free roll and some feta cheese.

Calories 396 kcals | **Serves** 2

Minestrone

The Italian classic works just as well with brown rice as with pasta. Always rinse rice well before cooking to get rid of the starch that can make it go gloopy.

25 g (1 oz) brown rice
1 teaspoon olive oil
Half a red onion, finely chopped
1 carrot, peeled and chopped into 1 cm (½ in) dice
1 courgette, chopped into 2 cm (¾ in) dice
4 tablespoons tomato passata
Salt and black pepper

To serve, per person:
3 black pepper oatcakes
30 g (1 oz) soft goats' cheese

1 Rinse the brown rice thoroughly and put it in a pan. Cover it well with water, bring it to the boil and cook until the rice is just beginning to soften – probably about 15–20 minutes. Then drain the rice and rinse it under a cold tap.

2 Warm the olive oil in a heavy saucepan. Add the onion and cook over a medium heat, allowing the onion to soften but not burn – keep an eye on it and stir it well, adding a little water towards the end of the time if it seems to be catching.

3 Add the chopped carrot to the pan, stir it around, and then add the chopped courgette. Cook for a minute or so, and then add the cooked rice, the passata and enough water to cover everything well. Season with salt and pepper and bring to the boil.

4 Reduce the heat and simmer for 15 minutes or until the rice is cooked and the carrots are tender. Serve, accompanied by the oatcakes and goats' cheese.

Tangy hummous with crudités

Why does anyone buy packaged hummous when the homemade
version is so easy to prepare and so much tastier? It beats us!
Make the hummous at least an hour before you want to eat.
Cover the bowl with clingfilm and keep in the fridge.

200 g (7 oz) chickpeas
1 small garlic clove, finely chopped
2 level teaspoons tahini paste
2 teaspoons olive oil
Juice of 1 large lemon
Black pepper

For the crudités:
3–4 carrots, peeled and cut into sticks
A quarter of a cucumber, deseeded and cut into sticks
6 spring onions, trimmed
A few raw cauliflower florets

1 Drain and rinse the chickpeas and put them in a pan with some
   water. Cook over a medium heat for about 3 minutes to warm
   them through. Drain, reserving some of the liquid, and transfer
   them to a blender.

2 Add the garlic to the blender. Stir the jar of tahini well, and add
   2 teaspoons to the blender. Add the olive oil and lemon juice
   and blitz until smooth; it may be necessary to add a little of the
   reserved chickpea cooking liquid to get the right consistency.
   Spoon the hummous into a bowl and allow it to cool down.

3 Serve the cooled hummous with the crudités.

TIP
This is great for a packed lunch – just wrap up the crudités and put
the hummous into a sealable container rather than a bowl while it
cools down.

LUNCHES
Calories 400 kcals | **Serves** 1

North Indian carrot salad with cashew nuts in a baked potato

It's got very few ingredients but this carrot salad is utterly moreish. Served in a potato, it makes a nourishing, filling and extremely tasty lunch.

1 x 200 g (7 oz) baking potato
6 cashew nuts
2 medium–large carrots
1 tablespoon sesame oil
1 teaspoon whole black mustard seeds
Salt

1 Wash the potato and stab it several times with a fork or sharp knife. Put it in a microwave and cook it for 4 minutes at 800 watts. Turn it over, and cook for a further 4 minutes or so (adjust times for individual microwaves) until it is cooked right through. Alternatively, bake the potato in the oven. Preheat the oven to 200°C (400°F), Gas mark 6, and wash the potato skin. Cut a line round the middle of the potato and pierce it several times with a fork. Place it on a baking sheet and bake for 1–1½ hours or until the potato is soft.

2 While the potato is cooking, prepare the salad. Split the cashew nuts and put a small frying pan over a medium to high heat. When it is hot, add the cashews and toss them in the pan to dry roast them briefly, until they just begin to colour. Set them to one side.

3 Peel the carrots. Using a coarse grater (or food processor disc), grate them into a bowl. Add a little salt, and stir. Heat the oil in the frying pan and add the mustard seeds. They will start to pop and split very quickly; take the pan off the heat when they do and empty the warm oil and seeds into the grated carrot. Stir everything together well, then put the carrot onto a serving plate and garnish with the cashew nuts. Serve immediately, accompanied by the baked potato.

Calories 395 kcals | **Serves** 1

Roasted beetroot and feta salad

The sweetness of the beetroot contrasts with the saltiness of the cheese and the tanginess of the lemon, making a very satisfying dish that tastes much more calorific than it is.

3 small–medium beetroot (raw)
Mixed salad leaves or lettuce
100 g (3½ oz) feta cheese
2 teaspoons Lemon Dressing (see page 60)
Salt and black pepper

1 Preheat the oven to 200°C (400°F), Gas mark 6.

2 Gently clean the raw beets but do not peel or top and tail them. Wrap each one in foil, sealing the little packages well, and put them on a baking sheet. Bake until they give slightly when you squeeze the packets. Test that they are cooked by unwrapping one and sticking a knife in – it should go in gently but the beetroot should not be mushy; the skin should also wrinkle slightly. Carefully unwrap the beetroot and let them cool a little. Then slide the skins off; they should come off easily but may need to be helped with a knife. Put the peeled beetroot to one side.

3 Pile the salad leaves on a plate. Chop the beetroot and scatter the pieces over the leaves. Rinse the feta cheese and pat it dry, then crumble the feta over the beetroot. Drizzle the lemon dressing over the salad and season with black pepper – the feta will still be quite salty, so test before adding any more. Serve immediately.

TIP
For a packed lunch, take the chopped beetroot in a separate container and add it to the rest of the salad just before serving.

Calories 400 kcals | **Serves** 1

New potato salad with cherry tomatoes, herbs and smoked mackerel

'Potatoes? Aren't they banned on most diets?' you may ask. But we see no reason to cut out such a good source of vitamin C, potassium and iron. They're the perfect complement to a piece of smoked fish that's full of healthy oils.

125 g (4 oz) small new potatoes
3 tablespoons low-fat mayonnaise
5 spring onions, finely chopped
A handful of fresh chives, chopped
A small handful of fresh parsley, chopped
3–4 sprigs of fresh basil, torn
5 cherry tomatoes, halved
A small fillet of smoked mackerel with black pepper,
    about 40 g (1 ½ oz)
Salt and black pepper

1 Fill a pan with water, add a little salt and the potatoes, and bring to the boil. Cook until the potatoes are tender – the timing will depend on the size of the potatoes; test them with a fork – and then drain them well. Cut any large potatoes in half while they are still warm and put them all in a bowl. Add the mayonnaise and black pepper to taste, and stir gently until the mayo and potatoes are thoroughly mixed. Set the bowl aside for the salad to cool a little.

2 Add the spring onions, chives and parsley. Stir once more, then gently stir in the halved cherry tomatoes and torn basil.

3 Remove the skin from the mackerel fillet, flake the mackerel flesh, then scatter it into the salad and stir it gently once more. Check the seasoning and serve immediately.

TIP
For a packed lunch, take the tomatoes, basil and mackerel separately and add them just before serving.

Chickpea salad with tuna, red onion and garlic croûtons

Served warm or cold, this is a filling and very nutritious lunch that packs all the food groups and plenty of flavour as well.

200 g (7 oz) chickpeas
1 x 80 g (3 oz) can tuna in spring water or brine
Half a small red onion, finely chopped
A small bunch of fresh parsley, chopped
A few leaves of fresh coriander, chopped (optional)
2 teaspoons Lemon or Garlic Dressing (see page 60)
Black pepper
Mixed salad leaves or lettuce

For the croûtons:
1 slice of wheat-free bread
1 small garlic clove
½ teaspoon olive oil

1 Drain and rinse the chickpeas and put them in a pan with some water. Simmer over a medium heat for about 3 minutes to warm them through. Drain well.

2 Drain the tuna, rinse it if it has been canned in brine, and flake it into a bowl. Add the chickpeas and red onion and stir everything together. Add the parsley and coriander leaves (if using). Add the dressing and some black pepper, and stir together. Put a good helping of salad leaves on a plate, and tip the chickpea and tuna on top.

3 For the croûtons, toast a slice of wheat-free bread until golden. Rub one side with the clove of garlic and drizzle it with the olive oil. Cut it into cubes and scatter over the salad. Serve immediately.

TIP
If taking as a packed lunch, it may be more convenient to replace the croûtons with an ordinary slice of wheat-free toast.

Calories 400 kcals | **Serves** 1 generously

Crunchy coleslaw with a wheat-free roll

No doubt you've tasted coleslaw before – but not like this. It's crunchy and creamy with lots of different textures and flavours. This is a recipe you'll use time and again.

Half a head of fennel (optional – if omitted, add more carrot)
3 spring onions
100 g (3½ oz) white cabbage, shredded
1 large carrot, peeled and grated
3 tablespoons low-fat mayonnaise
1 teaspoon Dijon mustard
Salt and black pepper
2 walnut halves
1 brown wheat-free roll, to serve

1 Take the outside layer off the fennel (if using) and chop the rest of the bulb finely, then add to a bowl. Trim the spring onions and cut them into short lengths. Put them in the bowl with the rest of the vegetables, and mix everything together.

2 Put the mayonnaise in a separate bowl and stir in the mustard; blend them together and then add the mayo to the large bowl. Stir everything thoroughly to lightly coat the vegetables with the dressing, and season well with salt and black pepper.

3 Just before serving, chop the walnuts and scatter them over the coleslaw. Serve with a brown wheat-free roll – you shouldn't need any spread on it.

TIP
If the coleslaw is to be a packed lunch, take the walnuts separately.

Feta dip with crudités

Imagine you are sailing across azure sea around the Greek islands. Your yacht moors at a tiny harbour where there is a taverna. You sit down at a table and they bring you a dish of this feta dip. Enjoy!

100 g (3½ oz) feta cheese
3 tablespoons 0%-fat Greek yogurt
1 small garlic clove, crushed
A squeeze of lemon juice
1 teaspoon olive oil
Black pepper

For the crudités:
2 carrots
4–5 celery sticks
5 spring onions
A quarter of a cucumber

1 Rinse the feta under running water, pat it dry and crumble it into a bowl. Mash with a fork, then add the yogurt and mix it in well, still mashing until the texture is much smoother.

2 Add the garlic, lemon juice and olive oil to the bowl. Work the ingredients together with a fork until they are all well mixed and any remaining pieces of feta have broken up. Add lots of black pepper and stir well. Transfer the dip to a serving bowl and put it in the fridge for a little to allow the flavours to mingle.

3 Prepare the crudités. Peel the carrots and cut them into sticks. Remove the strings from the outside of the celery sticks and chop them in half, and trim the spring onions. Cut the cucumber into strips and remove the seeds.

4 Serve the dip with the crudités; just wrap the crudités in clingfilm to take them as part of a packed lunch.

Lentil, tomato and goats' cheese salad

Choose a crumbly, rather than a creamy, goats' cheese
(see page 73). A chunk about the size of a man's thumb
will add plenty of tangy flavour to this filling salad.

50 g (2 oz) Puy lentils
1 bay leaf
1 teaspoon olive oil
2 small tomatoes
Half a small red onion, finely chopped
A handful of fresh parsley
Mixed salad leaves or lettuce
50 g (2 oz) goats' cheese
A squeeze of lemon juice
Salt and black pepper

1 Check the lentils for any small stones, then rinse them and put
   them in a pan of water. Add the bay leaf. Put the pan over a high
   heat and bring to the boil, then reduce the heat and simmer for
   about 20 minutes or until the lentils are soft.

2 Discard the bay leaf and rinse the cooked lentils briefly; they
   should still be slightly warm. Put them in a bowl, add a little salt
   and black pepper, and then add the oil. Stir and set to one side.
   Quarter the tomatoes and remove the seeds. Chop the tomato
   pieces and add them to the bowl along with the onion and parsley.
   Mix everything together.

3 Put some salad leaves on a plate and pile the lentil salad on top.
   Crumble the goats' cheese over the lentils and add a quick squeeze
   of lemon juice and a little more seasoning if necessary. Serve
   immediately.

TIP
If this is to be a packed lunch, take the goats' cheese separately and
add it just before you eat.

Calories 390 kcals | **Serves** 1 generously

Celeriac remoulade with a baked potato

If you are not familiar with celeriac, do give it a try. It usually features on the menus of all the top French restaurants, and for good reason.

2 tablespoons low-fat mayonnaise
2 teaspoons Dijon mustard
2 anchovy fillets (canned in oil)
1 teaspoon capers
Zest of 1 lemon
200–250 g (7–8 oz) celeriac root
1 x 200 g (7 oz) baking potato
Salt and black pepper

1 Put the mayonnaise and mustard in a large bowl. Blot the anchovy fillets on kitchen paper to remove any excess oil, then shred them into the mixture and break them up well with a fork. Roughly chop the capers and add them to the bowl. Then, add the lemon zest. Stir everything together, and season to taste.

2 Put a pan of water onto the boil and prepare the celeriac. Trim off the peel and any roots and chop the celeriac into long pieces. Cut these pieces into fine julienne strips with a sharp knife, or use a food processor. Plunge the strips into the pan of boiling water. Let the pan return to the boil and cook for 1 minute, then remove from the heat and drain the celeriac in a sieve. Rinse it under a cold tap and shake it well to dry thoroughly (if necessary, dry it in a tea towel). Put the blanched celeriac into the bowl of dressing and turn it well to mix. Cover the bowl and refrigerate for 1 hour.

3 Cook the potato just before you are ready to eat, following the instructions on page 49. Serve with the celeriac.

Calories 430 kcals I **Serves** 1

Prawn and melon salad

Now for a real taste of luxury! Choose nice big meaty, fresh prawns, and sniff the melon before you buy to make sure it is aromatically sweet and ripe.

125 g (4 oz) cooked prawns
Half a small galia melon
1 celery stick
1 tablespoon low-fat mayonnaise
1 tablespoon low-fat natural yogurt
1 teaspoon wholegrain mustard
Salt and black pepper
1 brown wheat-free roll, to serve

1 Rinse the prawns and dry them thoroughly, then put them in a large bowl. Remove the seeds from the melon half and use a spoon or a melon baller to scoop out the flesh – or cut the melon into slices, remove the skin and chop the flesh into 1 cm (½ in) cubes. Add the melon to the bowl. Remove the strings from the celery stick, chop it finely and add it to the bowl, too.

2 Mix the mayonnaise, yogurt and mustard in a separate container, then add this dressing to the bowl and mix everything together thoroughly. Cover the bowl and set a side in a cool place for 30 minutes before serving. Check the seasoning and add some black pepper. Serve with a brown wheat-free roll – you shouldn't need any spread on it.

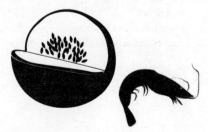

Hot chicken-strip salad

This is much better warm from the pan so if you are not near a kitchen, swap it for a lunch that has roughly the same calories and make this next time you are able to cook.

Mixed salad leaves or lettuce
2 teaspoons Classic Vinaigrette Dressing (see opposite)
2 small shallots, finely chopped
1 large tomato, finely chopped
1 skinless chicken breast, about 200 g (7 oz)
1 teaspoon olive oil
A sprig of fresh thyme
Salt and black pepper

1 Prepare the salad first, because the chicken does not take long to cook. Toss the salad leaves with the dressing and scatter over the chopped shallots and tomatoes.

2 Cut the chicken breast width-ways into slices no wider than 1 cm (½ in); if any slices are very thick, cut them in half along their length. Warm the oil in a nonstick frying pan over a medium heat and add the chicken. Cook for 3–4 minutes, stirring, or until the pieces are starting to brown well and the edges are beginning to crisp up.

3 Scatter the thyme leaves over the chicken, turn the strips once more in the pan and check that they are cooked and tender. Take the pan off the heat and arrange the chicken over the salad. Season to taste with a little salt and black pepper, and serve immediately.

TIP
Add this recipe to your online diary at The Biggest Loser Club (www.biggestloserclub.co.uk), as used by The Biggest Loser contestants, for your daily calorie count.

SALAD DRESSINGS

These recipes give larger quantities than should be used at any one time. Use the serving sizes given in the recipes and keep the rest of the dressing in the fridge, using it within a week. Always shake well before use. Note: you'll need 5 clean jars with tightly fitting lids. Old jam jars or mayonnaise jars would do fine.

Shallot dressing

5 teaspoons olive oil
2 teaspoons balsamic vinegar
1 small shallot
Salt and black pepper

1 Get a small clean jar and put the oil and vinegar into it. Add a pinch of salt and a slightly larger pinch of black pepper. Peel and chop the shallot finely and add it to the jar. Seal the jar, making sure the top is firmly on, and shake well before using.

Calories 215 kcals (per jar) | **Makes** 8 x 1 teaspoon servings

Classic vinaigrette dressing

1 Make this in the same way as the shallot dressing, but replace the shallot with 1 teaspoon Dijon mustard.

Calories 205 kcals (per jar) | **Makes** 7–8 x 1 teaspoon servings

Thyme dressing

1 Make the classic dressing and add 1 teaspoon fresh thyme leaves before shaking the jar.

Calories 205 kcals (per jar) | **Makes** 8 x 1 teaspoon servings

Lemon dressing

5 teaspoons olive oil
2 teaspoons lemon juice
Black pepper

1 Put the oil and lemon juice in a small clean jar. Add a pinch of black pepper. Seal the jar, making sure the top is firmly on, and shake well before using.

Calories 210 kcals (per jar) | **Makes** 7 x 1 teaspoon servings

Garlic dressing

1 garlic clove
5 teaspoons olive oil
2 teaspoons balsamic vinegar
¼ teaspoon Dijon mustard

1 Peel the garlic. Put the oil and vinegar in a small jug or bowl and crush the garlic into it. Stir well, crushing the garlic further with the spoon, and then pass the dressing through a sieve into a small jar; discard the pieces of garlic left in the sieve. Add the mustard, seal the jar, shake well and use.

Calories 205 kcals (per jar) | **Makes** 7–8 x 1 teaspoon servings

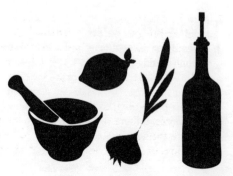

Calories 400 kcals | **Serves** 2

Chicken and pepper casserole

If you're making this for someone who is not watching their
weight, you could add some tagliatelle as an accompaniment.
But you will feel perfectly full after taking in 357 kcal
(per 100 g/3½ oz serving of pasta) fewer than them.

1 teaspoon olive oil
Half a large red onion, chopped
2 skinless chicken breasts, about 225 g (7½ oz) each
300 ml (½ pint) chicken stock (made using no more than half a stock cube)
   or water
1 large red pepper, deseeded and chopped into 2 cm (¾ in) chunks
1 large yellow pepper, deseeded and chopped into 2 cm (¾ in) chunks
100 ml (3½ fl oz) tomato passata with herbs
1 tablespoon tomato purée
150 g (5 oz) mushrooms, chopped

To serve:
Mixed salad leaves or lettuce
2 teaspoons Classic Vinaigrette Dressing (see page 59)

1 Put the oil in a heavy saucepan with a lid, and warm it over a
   medium heat. Add the onion and cook gently for 5 minutes. Cut
   each chicken breast into 4 pieces and add to the pan. Allow each
   side of the chicken pieces to cook slightly, then add the stock.

2 Add the peppers, passata and the tomato purée and stir everything
   together. Bring to the boil, then lower the heat and simmer, partly
   covered, for 30 minutes. Check several times that there is still
   enough liquid – add a little water if it seems to be cooking away –
   and stir to make sure nothing sticks.

3 Add the mushrooms to the pan and continue to cook for a further
   20 minutes. If there still seems to be a lot of liquid in the casserole,
   increase the heat and allow it to boil for a few minutes. Serve with a
   large bowl of salad leaves, tossed with the classic dressing.

Calories 400 kcals | **Serves 1**

Omelette with soft goats' cheese and a tomato salad

This omelette is not for sharing. Lay out your best cutlery, light a candle and serve on a bone china plate. It deserves it!

For the salad:
3 tomatoes
4 black olives
2 teaspoons Classic Vinaigrette Dressing (see page 59)

For the omelette:
25 g (1 oz) soft, crumbly goats' cheese
2 large eggs
½ teaspoon olive oil spread
Salt and black pepper

1 Make the salad first. Slice the tomatoes finely and put them on a plate. Slice the olives and scatter them over the tomatoes. Drizzle it all with the vinaigrette dressing and set the plate to one side.

2 Crumble the goats' cheese and set it to one side too. Then crack the eggs into a bowl and beat them together with a little salt, some black pepper and a teaspoon of water.

3 Put the olive oil spread in a small nonstick frying pan over a medium heat. When it begins to froth, pour the eggs into the pan. Swirl them around and let them cook for a few seconds then stir them gently, drawing the cooking egg in from the outside towards the centre. Tilt the pan and let any uncooked liquid run out to the edges. The egg will soon begin to set; stop stirring when it does.

4 Scatter the goats' cheese over the top, keeping it away from the edge, and continue cooking for another minute or so. Fold the omelette over and slide it onto a plate. Serve immediately, with the tomato salad.

Calories 375–415 kcals depending on the weight of the tuna steak | **Serves 1**

Grilled tuna steak

Chefs sear the outside of tuna steaks and serve them still pink and raw in the middle, but do yours however you like it best.

1 x fresh tuna steak, about 150–200 g (6–7 oz)
1 large garlic clove
3 sprigs of fresh thyme
1 shallot
Juice of half a lemon
1 tablespoon balsamic vinegar
2 teaspoons olive oil
Salt and black pepper

To serve:
Rocket leaves
Mixed salad leaves or lettuce
2 tablespoons low-fat mayonnaise

1 Rinse the tuna steak and pat it dry, then prepare a marinade. Crush the garlic into a glass or ceramic dish and add the leaves from the thyme stalks. Add the shallot and lemon juice – don't throw away the squeezed lemon, though – then add the vinegar and a little black pepper. Rub the tuna in the marinade, turn it over and spoon some marinade over it so that it is well coated. Cover the dish with clingfilm and leave in the fridge for an hour or so.

2 Make up a large rocket and green leaf salad, and prepare some lemon mayonnaise by blending a little zest from the squeezed lemon with the low-fat mayonnaise in a small side dish.

3 Put a ridged griddle pan or heavy-bottomed frying pan over a high heat and when it is really hot, add the olive oil. Once the oil is smoking, lift the tuna out of the marinade and shake off the excess. Cook it quickly on both sides, searing it until it is done to your taste (how long this takes will depend on how thick it is). Season and serve immediately, accompanied by the green salad and lemon mayo.

Aubergine curry with green beans and cucumber raita

Who says curry has to be served with rice or naan? This one works well with green beans and a raita, and the aubergine chunks give it a lovely meaty texture.

1 large aubergine, about 500 g (1 lb)
5 tablespoons tomato purée
1 tablespoon vegetable oil
1 large onion
1 teaspoon paprika
1 teaspoon garam masala
1 small red chilli (or to taste)
100 g (3 ½ oz) French beans, to serve

For the raita:
Half a cucumber
250 g (8 oz) low-fat natural yogurt
½ teaspoon ground cumin

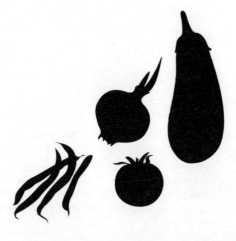

1 First cut the top off the aubergine, then chop it into 1–2 cm
(½–¾ in) cubes. Put the tomato purée in a bowl and mix with
2 tablespoons water. Pour the oil into a heavy-bottomed pan and
warm it over a medium to high heat. Peel the onion and halve it,
then chop one half well and slice the other into rings. Add all the
onion to the pan and cook it gently until it is soft and beginning
to change colour.

2 Add the paprika and garam masala, stir them in well and allow them
to cook for about a minute. Add the aubergine and the diluted
tomato purée, and stir well once more. Chop however much of the
chilli you want to use very finely and add it to the pan (don't forget
that chilli can sting, so wash your hands after chopping).

3 Lower the heat so that the curry is simmering and cover the pan.
Cook for 20 minutes or until the aubergine is soft, but check during
this time to make sure that the sauce has not cooked right away;
add more water if necessary, and give it a good stir to prevent it
from sticking. If there seems to be a lot of sauce, raise the heat for
the last few minutes so that some of it can cook off – this should
be quite a dry curry.

4 While the curry is cooking, make the raita. Grate the cucumber into
a bowl and then squeeze it, handful by handful, to release as much
water as possible. Drain and put the squeezed cucumber into a
clean bowl. Add the yogurt and cumin and stir it well; cover and
chill until the curry is cooked.

5 Towards the end of cooking, lightly boil or steam the green beans,
and serve them with the curry and the raita.

Calories 345–355 kcals | **Serves** 1

Aromatic salmon in a parcel

Lemon grass is a gift from the gods, turning a normal everyday salmon fillet into an exotic feast. Serve with steamed pak choi to emphasize the oriental theme, or choose any other green vegetables you like.

1 large salmon fillet, about 175 g (6 oz)
2 slices of lemon
2 slices of red onion
1 lemon grass stalk
1 bay leaf

To serve:
Pak choi, green vegetables or green salad (see below)
1 tablespoon soy sauce (optional)
1 teaspoon Lemon Dressing (see page 60), optional

1 Preheat the oven to 190°C (375°F), Gas mark 5. Rinse the salmon fillet and pat it dry. Take a large piece of foil and put the lemon and onion slices on it, then place the fish on top of them. Split the stalk of lemon grass and put a piece along each side of the fish, and rest the bay leaf on top. Now bring the edges of the foil up around the fish and over the top, and fold it together to make a slightly loose but well-sealed parcel.

2 Put the parcel in an ovenproof dish or roasting tin and cook for about 20 minutes, until the fish is cooked through and opaque; be careful when opening the parcel as hot steam will escape in a rush. Remove the bay leaf and lemon grass, and carefully lift the salmon off the lemon slices and onion; discard these.

3 Serve with either a large helping of steamed vegetables – pak choi (with soy sauce sprinkled on top), broccoli or mangetout – or with a large green salad dressed with a teaspoon of lemon dressing.

Calories 410 kcals (420 kcals for thighs) I **Serves** 1

Roast chicken pieces with lemon and herbs

The lemony, herby juices make this generous portion of roast chicken moist and flavourful. It would make a good Sunday dinner, and the rest of the family could have mashed potatoes alongside to beef it up a bit.

1½ teaspoons olive oil
I large skinless chicken breast, about 250 g (8 oz) or 2 large skinless
    chicken thighs, about 100 g (3½ oz) each
2 teaspoons dried mixed herbs
1 large lemon
Black pepper

To serve:
Mixed salad leaves or lettuce
2 small tomatoes, chopped
1 teaspoon Classic Vinaigrette Dressing (see page 59)

1 Preheat the oven to 200°C (400°F), Gas mark 6. Put 1 teaspoon of the olive oil in a baking dish and warm it in the oven. Rinse the chicken and pat it dry. Put the remaining oil on a plate, scatter the dried herbs over it, then roll the chicken in the oily-herby mixture.

2 Put the chicken in the baking dish. Cut the lemon in half, squeeze it and add the juice to the dish. Cut one of the lemon halves in quarters and tuck the pieces around the chicken. Put the dish back in the oven and bake for 15 minutes. Turn the chicken over and cook for a further 15 minutes. Turn them once more to brown them slightly, and cook them until they are done – when a knife goes in smoothly, the flesh is opaque with no tinge of pink and the juices run clear.

3 Put the chicken on a serving plate and discard the lemon pieces. Spoon a little of the juices in the baking dish over the chicken and serve immediately, accompanied by a salad with chopped tomatoes and a little classic dressing.

Calories 365 kcals | **Serves** 1

Stuffed pepper and courgette with a yogurt sauce

This is a big, tasty plate of food with a low calorie count that's also stacked with vitamins and minerals.

1 red pepper
1 medium–large courgette
2 teaspoons olive oil
Half a small red onion, chopped
1 garlic clove, chopped
250 g (8 oz) mushrooms, chopped
1 teaspoon tomato purée
3 teaspoons pine nuts
Salt and black pepper

For the sauce:
3 tablespoons low-fat natural yogurt
1 teaspoon Dijon mustard or a few drops of Tabasco sauce, to taste

1 Preheat the oven to 190°C (375°F), Gas mark 5. Cut the pepper, including the stalk, in half lengthways and remove the seeds and white membrane but leave the stalk on. Cut the stalk end off the courgette and cut it in half lengthways, too. Remove the middle using a teaspoon, but stop 1 cm (½ in) short of the cut end. Put the oil in a small dish and brush the pepper and courgette halves lightly with a little of it. Transfer them to a baking dish, cut side uppermost. Bake them in the oven for 15 minutes.

2 Meanwhile, prepare the stuffing. Drip the remaining oil into a nonstick frying pan over a medium heat. Add the chopped onion to the pan and cook gently for 5 minutes until it softens; don't let it catch. Then, add the garlic and cook for a further minute. Add the mushrooms. Increase the heat a little and cook the mushrooms until they are nice and soft – there should be very little liquid; cook a little longer if necessary. Then, add the tomato purée and stir. Remove the pan from the heat and take the baking dish out of the oven.

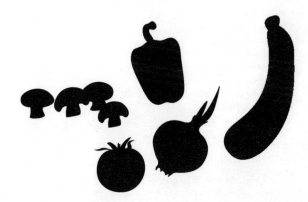

3 Put the pine nuts in a clean, dry pan and dry roast them, stirring, over a medium heat for a few seconds. They will quickly begin to colour; take the pan off the heat when they do. Carefully pile the cooked stuffing into the pepper and courgette halves, season with salt and pepper and scatter the pine nuts over them (if the oven has fierce top heat, add the pine nuts 10 minutes into the cooking time). Add a little boiling water around the vegetables – not more than 100 ml (3½ fl oz) – and return the baking dish to the oven. Cook for 20 minutes.

4 While the vegetables are cooking, mix the yogurt and Dijon mustard or Tabasco sauce together in a small bowl. When cooked, carefully lift the stuffed vegetables onto a serving plate – the water should all have evaporated – and add any filling which has fallen out. Serve with the yogurt sauce on the side.

DINNERS

Calories 435 kcals | **Serves** 1

Chicken stir-fry with oriental vegetables and cashew nuts

Stir-fries are only high in calories if you drown them in oil. The trick is to keep everything moving so that it doesn't get a chance to stick or burn, even when there's only a little oil.

1 skinless chicken breast, about 125 g (4 oz)
A dash of soy sauce
Half a red pepper
4 spring onions
1 head of pak choi
8 cashew nuts
1 garlic clove, finely chopped
1 cm (½ in) piece of fresh root ginger, finely chopped
1 tablespoon vegetable or sesame oil

1 Cut the chicken into pieces no larger than 1.5 cm (¾ in), and put them in a bowl. Sprinkle a little soy sauce over them and turn them so that they are well coated. Cover the bowl and set it to one side.

2 Prepare the vegetables. Chop the pepper into fine strips and cut the spring onions diagonally, including some of the greener part. Cut the pak choi into quarters. Carefully split the cashews in half.

3 Put a nonstick wok over a high heat and add the oil. Once the oil is really hot, add the chicken and cook for about 3 minutes, stirring well, until it is beginning to colour up nicely. Remove it from the wok with a slotted spoon and put it to one side on a plate. Add the pepper, spring onions, ginger and garlic and cook for a couple of minutes, still stirring, and then return the chicken and its juices to the wok. Add the pak choi and cook everything for a couple more minutes. Then add the cashews, stir to mix and serve immediately.

Prawns in garlicky tomato sauce

This tastes like catch of the day in Andalusia. Listen hard and you might hear the sound of gentle waves rolling up the beach and crickets chirping in the grass.

250 g (8 oz) raw king prawns
2 teaspoons olive oil
1 garlic clove, finely chopped
A little fresh chilli to taste or ¼ teaspoon cayenne pepper (optional)
4 tablespoons tomato passata
A squeeze of lemon
Salt and black pepper

To serve:
Mixed salad leaves or lettuce
A handful of basil leaves
2 teaspoons Classic Vinaigrette Dressing (see page 59)

1 Rinse the prawns in a sieve and shake them dry. Warm the olive oil in a frying pan over a medium heat. Add the garlic to the pan and cook it for a few seconds. If you are using fresh chilli, chop it finely and add it as well (it is a good idea to wash your hands after chopping chillies as the juice can sting sensitive areas such as lips and eyes).

2 Add the prawns to the pan and cook for 1–2 minutes; they will start to give off liquid. Put the passata in the pan, together with the cayenne pepper (if using), and cook everything over a high heat until the sauce is reduced by about half, which will probably take about 5 minutes. Add a pinch of salt, a little black pepper and stir everything together. Just before serving, squeeze some lemon juice over the prawns.

3 Serve with a large green salad scattered with the basil leaves and drizzled with the classic dressing.

Roasted vegetables with grilled goats' cheese

You can play mix and match with the vegetables without changing the calorie count significantly (as long as you avoid root vegetables). Swap one of the carrots for a small courgette cut into chunks, and if your peppers are on the small side, throw in a few cherry tomatoes.

1 teaspoon olive oil, plus a little extra to drizzle
1 large red onion
2 carrots
1 red pepper
1 yellow pepper
1 teaspoon dried mixed herbs
1 slim roundel of goats' cheese, about 80 g (3 oz)
Salt and black pepper

1 Preheat the oven to 200°C (400°F), Gas mark 6. Put most of the oil in a large ovenproof dish and put it in the oven to warm. Peel the onion and cut it into quarters, then cut each quarter into three. Peel and chop the carrots, then deseed and chop the peppers.

2 Take the dish out of the oven and add the vegetables, then scatter the dried herbs over them. Stir well and put the dish back in the oven. Bake for 15 minutes, then stir again, making sure that nothing is sticking too badly. Cook for another 15 minutes, or until the vegetables are soft and crisping up a little.

GOATS' AND SHEEP'S CHEESE

Most large supermarkets carry a good range of goats' cheese, including crumbly roundels and logs, flavoured varieties, harder, mature cheeses that are ideal for grating, and soft, spreadable cheeses that are much like cream cheese. If you find most goats' cheese too strongly flavoured, go for a lighter chevre blanc. All types of goats' cheese melt nicely.

A nice mellow feta made from sheep's milk (check the label; they aren't all) is a great addition to salads, casseroles, sandwiches or wraps, and hard sheep's cheeses, such as pecorino, are a good substitute for Parmesan. Manchego, a strong, mature sheep's milk cheese from Spain, is a good choice, as is sheep's milk Roquefort and Murcia al vino. You can find most of these in your local cheese shop or supermarket. If mozzarella is more to your taste, go for Buffalo milk varieties, which are soft and flavourful.

3 Now grill the goats' cheese (if the oven and grill are combined, take the vegetables out of the oven and keep them warm by covering the dish with a cloth). Preheat the grill to high. Put a square of foil on the work surface and unwrap the slice of cheese on top of it. Drizzle a little oil onto the cheese and season with black pepper. Put it under the grill until the top of the cheese begins to brown – this will probably take less than a minute.

4 Put the roasted vegetables on a warmed plate. Carefully remove the cheese from the foil using a fish slice and put it on top of the vegetables; season to taste and serve immediately.

Calories 360–370 kcals | **Serves** 1

Fish plaki

This Greek favourite is best made with a very fresh piece of fish.
It's a good dish to order in restaurants on holiday because it's
low-cal enough to keep you in swimwear shape.

2 teaspoons olive oil, plus a little extra for drizzling
1 onion
1 small–medium carrot
1 medium–large courgette
A sprig of fresh thyme, leaves only
1 bay leaf
250 g (8 oz) cod loin or similar fillet of white fish
Black pepper
Green vegetables or green salad (see below), to serve

1 Preheat the oven to 190°C (375°F), Gas mark 5. Heat the olive oil
in a large nonstick frying pan. Peel and chop the onion and carrot
finely – none of the vegetable pieces should be bigger than 1 cm
(½ in) – and add them to the pan. Cook for 2–3 minutes until the
onion is transparent. Chop the courgette and add this too. Cook for
another 3–4 minutes, until the vegetables are beginning to soften.

2 While the vegetables are cooking, drizzle a little oil on a baking
dish just slightly larger than the fish fillet and rub it around with
kitchen paper. Put the partly cooked vegetables into the baking
dish in an even layer and scatter the thyme leaves over them, then
add the bay leaf and black pepper. Put the fish fillet on top of the
vegetables, with the skin side uppermost. Add about 50 ml (2 fl oz)
water to the dish and put it into the oven. Bake for 20 minutes and
then check how the fish is cooking. Lift it up, give the vegetables
a stir and replace the fish. Cook for a further 5–10 minutes, until
the fish flakes easily.

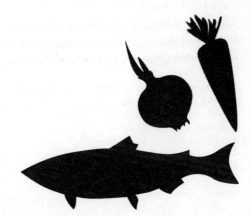

3 Lift the fish carefully onto a warmed serving plate. Remove the
   bay leaf, and then lift the vegetables out with a slotted spoon and
   arrange them next to the fish. Pour a tablespoon of the juices on
   top of the fish and serve immediately. Accompany with either a
   large helping of steamed vegetables – broccoli or mangetout are
   particularly good – or with a large green salad dressed with a
   teaspoon of Classic Vinaigrette Dressing (see page 59).

Salade Niçoise

You'll find a different version of this salad in every café along the French Riviera. There's a good reason why it's become a classic – it tastes great!

1 large egg
1 x 80 g (3 oz) can tuna in spring water or brine
Mixed salad leaves or lettuce
A quarter of a cucumber
A small bunch of fresh basil
3 small tomatoes
6 spring onions
8 black olives
10 fine green beans
3 anchovy fillets (optional)
3 teaspoons Classic Vinaigrette Dressing (see page 59)
Salt and black pepper

1 Hard-boil the egg – boil it for 10 minutes in salted water, then drain and allow it to cool in fresh water.

2 Drain the can of tuna, and rinse it if it was canned in brine. Arrange lots of salad leaves on a large plate. Cut the cucumber into rounds (peel it if you wish) and put them on top, then scatter a few basil leaves over and mix everything together. Spread the mixed salad over the plate.

3 Quarter the tomatoes and remove the seeds, slice the spring onions and cut the olives into chunks. Top and tail the beans and cut them into 2 cm (¾ in) lengths. Distribute the tomatoes, onions, olives and beans evenly on top of the salad leaves. Flake the tuna and scatter it over the plate. Then carefully peel the egg and cut it into quarters; place those on the plate as well. Blot the anchovies on kitchen paper, then break them into smaller pieces and add them too. Drizzle the dressing over everything, check the seasoning and serve immediately.

Grilled mushrooms with spinach and cheese

Look for meaty mushrooms that are at least 8 cm (3½ in) in diameter for a light but filling main course dish.

100 g (3½ oz) baby spinach leaves
1 garlic clove, chopped
1 teaspoon olive oil
1 small–medium red onion, or half a large one, finely chopped
3 large flat mushrooms, peeled and stalks removed
30 g (1 oz) soft goats' cheese or feta (see page 73)
Black pepper

To serve:
Mixed salad leaves or lettuce
3 teaspoons Shallot Dressing (see page 59)

1 Wash the spinach and squeeze the leaves dry, then chop them up. Put the spinach and garlic in a pan over a medium heat until the spinach has wilted. Drain well and set to one side.

2 Heat the olive oil in a small nonstick frying pan and gently cook the onion until it has softened and is just beginning to brown, about 5 minutes. Preheat the grill to high while the onion is cooking.

3 When the onion is just beginning to colour, add the drained spinach and garlic to the pan and cook them together until the spinach has warmed through, and any remaining liquid has cooked off.

4 Put the mushrooms on a baking sheet. Using a spoon, divide the spinach and onion mixture between the three mushrooms, covering as much of the flat surface as possible. Crumble the cheese over the top, and add a final sprinkling of black pepper. Put the mushrooms under the grill and cook for 5–6 minutes, or until the topping is beginning to brown nicely. Serve immediately, accompanied by a large green salad tossed with shallot dressing.

Calories 400 kcals | **Serves** 1

Pan-fried crispy salmon with courgettes and lemon mayonnaise

Never tried courgette 'spaghetti'? It has a crispness that is a perfect counterpoint to the moist salmon and creamy mayo.

200 g (7 oz) courgettes (1 large one or 2 smaller ones)
1 teaspoon olive oil
1–2 teaspoons black pepper
1 x salmon fillet, about 150 g (5 oz), skin on or off

For the lemon mayonnaise:
2 teaspoons lemon juice
1 rounded teaspoon low-fat mayonnaise

1 Fill a bowl with water. Top and tail the courgette and, using a potato peeler, peel the courgette into strips and drop them in the water; discard the very middle if there are too many seeds. Set the bowl to one side.

2 Put a teaspoon of the lemon juice in a small bowl and add the mayonnaise. Blend them together well; the mixture may seem to curdle at first, but carry on until the lemon mayonnaise is smooth. Put a pan of water on the heat to boil.

3 Put the olive oil in a small frying pan and place it over a high heat. While it warms, put the other teaspoon of lemon juice on a plate and add the black pepper. Dry the salmon fillet on kitchen paper and then place it, skin side downwards (or the side where the skin would have been), on top of the lemon and black pepper. Move the fish around to coat as much of the skin as possible in the lemon-pepper mixture.

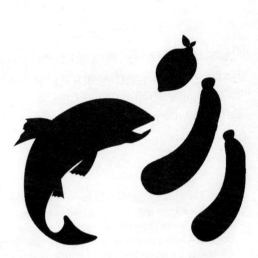

4 When the oil is hot, carefully put the fish in the pan, skin side down.
   Allow it to cook for 2 minutes, then turn it over carefully on to its
   side and cook for 2 minutes more. Repeat until all 4 sides of the
   slice of salmon have been cooked. Finally, turn it back onto the skin
   side for a further minute.

5 Just before the salmon is ready, drain the courgette strips and tip
   them into the boiling water. Cook them very briefly – no longer
   than 1 minute, then drain thoroughly. Take the salmon out of the
   pan and blot it on kitchen paper. Put the courgettes on a plate, top
   them with the crispy salmon and serve the lemon mayonnaise on
   the side.

Plum compôte with toasted almonds

This is as filling as a portion of plum crumble but with a third of the calories. Choose very ripe plums that don't need any sweetness added to them.

125 g (4 oz) red plums
8 whole almonds

1 Chop the plums roughly and remove the stones. Put them in a small pan with 2 tablespoons water, and place the pan over a medium heat. Cook the plums gently, stirring so they do not stick, until they begin to break up. Cook them for a couple more minutes, then pour them into a serving bowl and set to one side to cool – they taste good both hot or cold, but are best with the almonds when they are warm rather than hot.

2 Carefully split the almonds. Put a nonstick frying pan over a high heat. When the pan is hot, add the almond halves and stir them around. Take the pan off the heat as soon as the nuts begin to smell toasted, tip them on top of the plums and serve.

APPLE COMPÔTE

You can make a tasty apple compôte in a similar fashion. Peel and chop 2 dessert apples, dropping them into water. Drain most of the water away and add 1 tablespoon sultanas and 1 teaspoon raisins. Put the pan over a medium–hot heat. The apples will soon start to soften and release their juice; add ¼ teaspoon ground cinnamon when they do. Stir regularly – if it seems to be sticking, add a little more water – and cook until the apples are beginning to break down. Remove the pan from the heat and either serve immediately with 2 tablespoons 0%-fat Greek yogurt on the side, or allow to cool and eat later. Calories: 160.

DESSERTS
Calories 150 kcals I **Serves** 1

Pan-fried apples with cinnamon

Apple and cinnamon is a classic flavour combination that never dates. This is one of the few recipes in the book that requires butter rather than olive-oil spread – but be sparing.

1 sliver of butter, not more than 10 g (½ oz)
2 small dessert apples, peeled, cored and sliced
¼ teaspoon ground cinnamon

1 Put a small nonstick frying pan over a medium heat and melt the butter. Scatter the apples in the pan so that they form a single layer, as far as that is possible. Cook them gently for about 2–3 minutes until they are beginning to soften and brown (how long this takes will depend on the variety of apple used).

2 Scatter the cinnamon over the apples and turn them over carefully, using a fish slice. Cook the other sides for a couple of minutes, until they also begin to brown, and then slide them onto a plate and serve immediately.

TIP
Discover more delicious dessert recipes at The Biggest Loser Club (www.biggestloserclub.co.uk).

Fresh fruit salads

The art of a good fruit salad lies in gorgeous colours as well as flavours that complement each other. Each one of these is a thing of beauty that could grace any dinner party menu.

Green fruits

1 kiwifruit
5–6 green seedless grapes
1 small–medium green apple
2 tablespoons orange juice
2 tablespoons 0%-fat Greek yogurt

1 Peel the kiwifruit and chop it into a serving bowl. Slice the grapes in half and add them too, then cut the apple into quarters and remove the core (do not peel). Chop the apple into smaller pieces and add it to the bowl. Drizzle the orange juice over the fruit and stir everything together well. Serve, accompanied by the yogurt.

Calories 140 kcals | **Serves** 1

Red and black

50 g (2 oz) strawberries
100 g (3½ oz) blueberries
6–7 black grapes
2 tablespoons orange juice
1 watermelon slice

1 Wash and hull the strawberries, and chop them into halves. Put them in a serving bowl and tip in the blueberries. Then deseed and slice the grapes and add them to the bowl, followed by the orange juice. You can either use a spoon or melon baller to make even-sized balls of watermelon, or cut the melon into pieces; either way, remove as many seeds as possible. Then add the melon to the salad, stir well and serve.

Calories 140 kcals | **Serves** 1

Melon, grape and ginger

1 cm (½ in) piece of fresh root ginger, peeled
Half a large galia melon
A pinch of ground ginger (optional)
100 g (3½ oz) black grapes

1 Grate the fresh ginger into a small pan and add 4 tablespoons of
water. Put over a high heat and boil, reducing and concentrating the
liquid by at least half. Then pass it through a sieve into a container
and allow the ginger water to cool. Discard the ginger pieces.

2 Cut the melon into slices and remove the skin. Chop the flesh into
chunks, put them into a serving bowl and scatter a little ground
ginger over them if you want a stronger ginger flavour. Halve and
deseed the grapes and add them to the bowl. Pour over the ginger
water, stir everything together and serve.

Calories 155 kcals I **Serves** 1

Black and gold

1 orange
3 stoneless prunes
1 teaspoon raisins
1 date
2 tablespoons orange juice

1 Carefully peel the orange, removing as much of the white pith
as possible. Separate it into segments, halve them and put them
in a serving bowl. Cut the prunes in half and add them to the
bowl, then scatter the raisins over. Slice the date into rounds and
add those too. Finally, add the orange juice and mix everything
together. Cover the bowl with clingfilm and chill it in the fridge
for 30 minutes before serving.

Calories 155 kcals I **Serves** 1

Calories 205 kcals | **Serves** 1

Warm grilled peaches with pine nuts or almonds

Peaches are the taste of summer, and grilling intensifies their heady sweetness. Nuts are high-calorie, though, so measure or count them out carefully and don't sneak any extras.

2 ripe peaches
15 g (½ oz) pine nuts, or 8 blanched almonds

1 Preheat the grill to high. Carefully cut the peaches into halves and remove the stones. Put the halves in a small heatproof dish, cut side uppermost, and scatter the pine nuts over them (if you are using almonds, chop them first).

2 Put the dish under the grill and cook until the pine nuts or almonds are warm and turning golden brown – keep an eye on them, because this will happen quite quickly. Serve immediately.

Calories 180 kcals (190 kcals if using the dried fig) I **Serves** 1

Dried fruit salad

A sweet treat with loads of fibre to get your bowels working efficiently. Who needs shop-bought sweets, which are full of artificial colours and flavourings? This is tastier, healthier and bursting with natural goodness.

1 tea bag, preferably Earl Grey
8 dried apricots
2 unstoned prunes or 1 dried fig
1 tablespoon sultanas
2 teaspoons dried cranberries or blueberries
2 tablespoons 0%-fat Greek yogurt

1 Make a cup of tea with the tea bag (but don't add milk) and put 2 tablespoons of the tea in a bowl. Cut the apricots and prunes in half, and chop the fig finely if using. Add them to the bowl, then add the sultanas and berries. Stir well, cover the bowl and set it to one side for at least an hour, or refrigerate overnight. The dried fruit will absorb all or most of the liquid and become much more tender; if necessary, drain before serving with a little yogurt.

50-calorie snacks

Fresh fruit:
- 1 dessert apple
- 1 small pear
- 1 peach or nectarine
- 2 plums
- 2 clementines, tangerines or satsumas
- 3 fresh apricots
- A dessert bowl of strawberries, raspberries, blackberries or cherries – but served plain, with no cream, yogurt or sugar
- A small punnet of blueberries, weighing about 150 g (5 oz)
- A handful of grapes, weighing about 80 g (3 oz)

Dried fruit and nuts:
- 2 dates
- 4 large dried apricots
- A small handful of sultanas
- 2 brazil nuts
- 3 cashew nuts
- 6 hazelnuts
- 15 pistachios

Olives:
- 10 black olives in brine (rinse well), or 10 stuffed green olives
- 15 green (unstuffed) olives in brine

100-calorie snacks

Simple and straightforward:
- 1 banana
- 1 orange and 3 almonds
- 1 apple and 20 g (1 oz) feta cheese
- 1 black pepper oatcake with a sliver of feta
- 2 plain oatcakes
- 1 plain oatcake with 1 teaspoon of smooth peanut butter
- 1 slice of wheat-free toast with Marmite
- 125 g (4 oz) pot low-fat unsweetened natural yogurt
- 150 g (5 oz) pot 0%-fat Greek yogurt
- Crudités with a heaped tablespoon of Feta Dip (see page 54) or Hummous (see page 48)

Or try one of the following:

Tzatziki and crudités

Half a cucumber
A little crushed garlic
1–2 fresh mint leaves, chopped
100 g (3½ oz) 0%-fat Greek yogurt
Black pepper
Carrot and celery sticks, trimmed spring onions, chunks of fennel or more cucumber, to serve

1 Chop the cucumber well and put it in a bowl. Add the crushed garlic, the mint and the yogurt. Stir well, grind some black pepper over and serve with your vegetable crudités.

Calories 100 kcals | **Serves** 1

SNACKS

Frozen fruit salad

1 ripe mango
100 g (3½ oz) seedless black grapes

1 Peel and dice the mango, then spread the pieces on a baking sheet so that they do not touch. Transfer the sheet to the freezer until the mango is frozen solid. Carefully remove the mango from the baking sheet and store in a freezer box.

2 Rinse your black grapes and freeze those too. Take half the mango out of the freezer and half a portion of grapes, allow them to soften a little – and eat. Save the other half for another time.

Calories 125 kcals I **Serves** 1

Baked banana

1 large banana

1 Place the whole, unpeeled banana into an oven preheated to 180°C (350°F), Gas mark 4. Bake for 20–25 minutes until the skin goes black and the banana is soft; turn it over once during this time. Cut a slit along the length of the fruit and eat with a spoon.

Calories 125 kcals I **Serves** 1

More substantial snacks (about 225–250 calories)

- If you want something sweet, have one of the fruit desserts on pages 80–85 with a dollop of 0%-fat Greek yogurt.
- Carefully measure a 50 g (2 oz) chunk of your favourite goats' cheese and eat it with an apple, 80 g (3 oz) grapes or an oatcake. Don't cheat on the cheese quantity though.
- Have 1 slice of wheat-free toast with 3 level teaspoons of smooth peanut butter.
- Have 1 wheat-free brown roll with a scraping of olive-oil spread (or 1 teaspoon of low-fat mayonnaise), with a slice of chicken and a sliced tomato inside.

Or try one of the following:

Tapenade

150 g (5 oz) pitted black olives in brine
½ teaspoon dried mixed herbs
3½ teaspoons olive oil
25 g (1 oz) capers
Half a garlic clove, crushed
2 anchovy fillets

To serve:
5–6 celery sticks
2 carrots, cut into thick strips
1 oatcake

1 Drain and rinse the olives well. Put them in a bowl, scatter them
  with the dried herbs and drizzle them with half a teaspoon of the
  olive oil. Stir them together, then cover the bowl and set it to one
  side for an hour or more (overnight is fine).

2 Tip the olives into a food processor and add the capers, garlic and
  anchovy fillets. Finally add the remaining 3 teaspoons of olive oil
  and process the mixture until it is as smooth as you can get it.

3 Serve as a dip, with crudités and an oatcake.

Calories 225 kcals | **Serves** 2 (will keep overnight in the fridge)

Strawberry banana smoothie – and others…

150 g (5 oz) strawberries
1 banana
150 ml (¼ pint) natural low-fat yogurt
3 ice cubes

1 Wash and hull the strawberries, and chop them roughly. Peel and chop the banana and put the pieces in a blender, then tip in the strawberries and add the yogurt. Blend everything together and add a little water to thin the smoothie to the texture you prefer; blend it again. Put the ice cubes in a glass and pour the smoothie on top; serve immediately.

Other smoothies can be made in the same fashion. Try:
• 150 g (5 oz) raspberries and 100 g (3½ oz) blueberries with the yogurt (155 calories).
• 2 kiwifruit and an apple and yogurt – peel and chop the fruit first (215 calories).
• Peel and chop a ripe mango and blend that with the yogurt to make a mango lassi (255 calories).

Calories 225 kcals | **Serves** 1

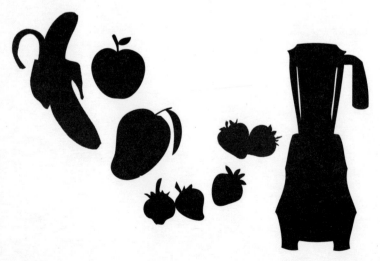

Olives with feta and herbs

125 g (4 oz) pitted black olives in brine
30 g (1 oz) feta cheese
½ teaspoon dried mixed herbs, or leaves from several sprigs of fresh thyme
A few dried chilli flakes (optional)
2 teaspoons olive oil
Black pepper

1 Rinse the olives well under cold water and put them in a bowl. Rinse the feta too, and then chop it into pieces. Add it to the bowl. Then scatter in the herbs and a few chilli flakes, if using, and add plenty of black pepper.

2 Pour the olive oil over the olives and cheese and carefully stir everything together. Cover and leave for at least 1 hour before serving, to give the different flavours time to work together. Pick at them throughout the day if you wish (using a cocktail stick or small fork will minimize messy hands).

Calories 245 kcals I **Serves** 1

Foods to avoid – and why

You may have noticed that certain foods are missing from the Beach Body Blitz plan. We'll be explaining some of these omissions in the next few pages, because it could be that you feel a whole lot better after avoiding them for a fortnight and might want to know why.

Overall, your system is getting a bit of a detox – a deep internal cleanse – to relieve pressure on all those congested organs, such as the liver and kidneys, and to eliminate any waste products that are clogging up the digestive system. The heavy, sugary, fat-laden meals and snacks full of artificial additives that we tend to favour in the Western world take their toll on our systems after a while, and start creating all kinds of unpleasant side effects.

These are the common signs of an overworked system:

- ☐ Excess gas and a bloated stomach, with either constipation or diarrhoea or both.
- ☐ Heartburn or acid reflux.
- ☐ Frequently having to get up in the night to urinate.
- ☐ Headaches.
- ☐ Cellulite on the thighs and upper arms.
- ☐ Skin rashes, a perpetually runny nose and other allergic-type symptoms.
- ☐ Bad breath and body odour.
- ☐ Dark circles under the eyes.
- ☐ Putting on fat round the abdomen.
- ☐ Women get more PMS and heavier periods.
- ☐ Swollen ankles and water retention.
- ☐ Cravings for sugary or fatty foods.
- ☐ Lowered immunity, so that you catch every cold and flu bug doing the rounds.
- ☐ Exhaustion!

If you ticked any of the boxes above it would be well worth you considering trying the Beach Body Blitz plan to cleanse your system.

If you've been overweight or obese for a while, you may suffer from several of these symptoms, and they're not fun. They can cause social embarrassment, force you to take days off work, and increase feelings of low self-esteem. Two weeks alone is not going to undo all the damage, but avoiding some of the worst-offending foods and drinks – the 'culprits' as we call them – during this period can go a long way to relieving pressure on your liver and letting it get on with its job of filtering out waste products for elimination. If you keep drinking lots of water throughout the day, you'll detox faster. You could also try drinking herbal teas (see varieties on page 104), which will support your efforts.

We're not promising that all your symptoms will be relieved completely by the end of the two-week plan, but they should have improved significantly. After that, if you reintroduce foods gradually, one at a time, you should be able to identify which food (or foods) was the worst culprit for you and consider whether to eliminate it from your diet long-term. None of the six culprits listed on pages 94–103 are essential to good health, so if you feel a lot better when you are not consuming them, it's a bit of a no-brainer.

SALT

Too much salt is bad for you. We need a little salt for the sodium it contains but if your entire diet is made up of junk food and ready meals, you could be consuming more than ten times as much as you need. This will be putting strain on your kidneys and could be responsible for symptoms such as water retention, frequent urination and dark circles under the eyes. There's also a clear link between salt intake and high blood pressure, which increases the risk of heart attacks and strokes. We've recommended using natural sea salt in the recipes, as it contains lots of useful minerals, but keep it to a minimum.

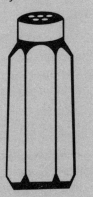

Less salt = less water retention
= less wobble.

Culprit no. 1 = sugar

You probably guessed this would be on the list. It's high in calories, it rots your teeth and it doesn't provide any useful nutrients that the body needs. But did you know that it is actually harmful to the rest of your system as well?

When you eat a sugary food, or drink a cup of tea with two sugars, the sugar is absorbed quickly into your blood stream. Your body produces a substance called insulin to help deal with this blood sugar peak. High insulin levels are not good news because they tell the body to store calories as fat, and they also prevent us from noticing the cut-off point when we feel full. The insulin mops up the sugar, our blood levels fall and we experience a dip in energy – and the desire to eat more sugar. That's right – eating sugary foods and drinks makes you want to eat more sugary foods and drinks.

Over time, if you keep eating lots of sugary foods and drinks, your system can become exhausted and stop producing enough insulin to cope with your sugar intake, and that's when you are at risk of developing diabetes. And diabetes is a bad disease to get. There's no cure, you have to change your lifestyle radically to cope with it, and some of its complications can be fatal.

That's not all. Eating lots of sugary foods can also harm your liver, which has to deal with all that excess insulin, and it can cause the growth of unhealthy bacteria in your gut, which can give you unpleasant digestive symptoms and prevent you from absorbing nutrients properly. None of which is good news for your general health.

In the past, some dieters have switched to artificial sweeteners, such as saccharine and sucralose, but we reckon that it's far better to wean yourself off sweet tastes altogether. Some studies have indicated that sweeteners might actually cause us to gain weight because our systems get confused when we taste sweetness, causing insulin to be released even though there is no sugar for it to work on. If you currently use sweeteners in tea or coffee, try to wean yourself off them gradually by cutting them into smaller and smaller pieces until they're virtually non-existent – and then stop completely.

SOME FOODS AND DRINKS CONTAINING SUGAR

- Alcohol (see pages 102–103)
- Biscuits
- Breads (some varieties)
- Breakfast cereals (many)
- Cakes
- Cappuccino mixes
- Cereal bars
- Chocolate
- Chutney and pickles
- Cook-in sauces
- Desserts
- Energy/sports drinks
- Fizzy drinks (apart from plain fizzy water)
- Honey
- Ice cream and ice lollies
- Jam/jelly
- Ketchup
- Low-fat products (such as yogurts)
- Marmalade
- Peanut butter
- Pies and flans
- Puddings
- Ready meals (even savoury ones)
- Salad dressings (shop-bought)
- Squash fruit drinks and cordials
- Sweets (everything from toffees to wine gums and boiled sweets)
- Table sauces (most)
- Yogurts (apart from natural ones)

It may not say 'sugar' on the label but watch out for its other names: glucose, dextrose, maltose, fructose, corn syrup, galactose, maltodextrin, lactose, sucrose, molasses, treacle, and anything ending in –ose or that has the word 'syrup' in it.

If you are a sugar junkie, this could be a hard addiction to quit, but take a look at your 'before' swimwear pictures and consider whether you can really face exposing that body to the world. There's no room on the Beach Body Blitz plan for chocolate (about 525 kcal per 100 g/3½ oz), sugary cereals (about 390 kcal per 100 g/3½ oz) or chocolate éclairs (396 kcal per 100 g /3½ oz). Each of them contains an entire meal's worth of calories. Put them in your mouth and you might as well apply them directly to your hips.

Deep down, every overweight person knows that the sugar's got to go!

Culprit no. 2 = wheat

Do you find that your stomach is much bigger at bedtime than it was when you got up in the morning? Has it ballooned? Are the buttons on your waistband straining?

If so, you are not alone. Lots of us get bloated during the day, for a number of different reasons. Some digestive diseases, such as irritable bowel syndrome, coeliac disease and Crohn's disease, have bloating as a side effect. It can be a symptom of something serious, and if bloating persists you should consult a doctor. But when you have two weeks to get into shape for the beach, it's worth cutting out all the types of food that can cause bloating – and one of the main culprits is wheat.

On its own, wheat is a perfectly nutritious grain, but the way we process and refine it in the modern world makes it harder for our bodies to digest. Most of us fail to absorb all the starch it contains, which then sits fermenting in the gut, producing gases and acids that can damage the lining of the gut. When you get into bed at night, press your lower abdomen and you may well hear the gurgling sounds inside and feel that there is gas in there. It's not all flab! Hooray! (If you are a deep sleeper, you may not know where that gas goes overnight, but chances are your partner does…)

If wheat is making you bloated, the good news is that two weeks without it will get rid of bloating and help the damaged gut walls begin to heal. In itself, wheat is not a high-calorie food but it tends to be eaten with high-calorie foods: bread with butter and jam, pizza with extra cheese and pepperoni, pasta with creamy sauce. It won't harm you to cut out wheat because you'll get the B vitamins and fibre it contains from other sources on the Beach Body Blitz eating plan. If you normally eat white bread and white flour products, they don't have any nutritional value anyway – you might as well be eating a piece of cardboard. Those all-important B vitamins and fibre are found in the husk of the grain, so you'll only get them in wholegrain products.

WHEAT SUBSTITUTES

Bread – major supermarkets and most health food shops sell wheat-free breads. Try a few until you find your favourite. (For online stockists, see page 223.)

Breakfast cereals – have whole oats instead, either cooked as porridge or in a wheat-free muesli (see page 40).

Pasta – supermarkets and health-food shops sell wheat-free pasta (just be careful not to overboil it or it goes gloopy). Alternatively, wholegrain brown rice is a good substitute.

Couscous – try quinoa, a nutritious grain with a similar texture.

Noodles – instead of your usual egg noodles, try rice noodles.

Biscuits and crackers – have a crunchy oatcake with tzatziki or tapenade on top (see page 83).

Pizza – not by any stretch of the imagination could pizza be called a health food, but if you simply can't live without it, make your own pizza base with wheat-free flour.

Sauces and gravy – thicken by boiling to reduce sauces rather than using flour or cornflour.

It can be tricky going permanently wheat-free in the modern world. You can't rush into a sandwich shop for a quick tuna-mayo baguette, and when eating out you have to question waiters about whether sauces were thickened with flour. But if you find you are not getting bloated any more after two wheat-free weeks on the Beach Body Blitz, it could be worth staying wheat-free longer-term. It's not just to make your stomach look flatter in clothes; your health could improve dramatically as well. Try a test after the holiday is over by eating a slice of wholegrain wheat bread and seeing how your gut reacts. If it isn't bloated a few hours later, then you can probably reintroduce wheat to your diet, but stick to brown, wholegrain bread and pasta rather than white, refined-flour products. It may be that there is another culprit causing your bloating – and there's a prime suspect on the next page.

Culprit no. 3 = dairy

Some of us have an intolerance to lactose,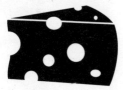
which is a sugar found in milk and milk products
(such as cream, ice cream, butter and cheese).
The problem is caused by us not having enough
lactase, the substance that digests milk sugar.
As we get older, we produce less and less of this lactase and
when we then polish off a cheese board our guts simply can't cope. The
lactose is not absorbed but moves down into the lower intestine where
unhealthy bacteria feed on it, causing gases to be produced, making
us bloated and flatulent. This is not what we want in our beachwear.

*Dairy products may or may not be causing your problems,
but by cutting down for a couple of weeks, you give your
liver and digestive system a rest – and cut a major source
of calories and fat from your diet.*

Do you have any idea how many calories are in a regular sized coffee-
shop latte made with whole milk? Around 200. What about a chunk
of Cheddar cheese the size of your thumb? Around 100. And 15 g
(½ oz) of butter – the amount you might spread on a couple of slices
of toast – adds 110 calories to your breakfast. They're also full of
saturated fats, the ones that are bad for your heart (see page 101).

Having said that, dairy products are an important source of calcium
so we don't want to cut them out entirely. Fortunately, they're not all
as bad as each other.

Cows' milk and cream are among the worst offenders, but people with
lactose intolerance often find they can eat goats' cheese without any
problems, so we've included some in the Beach Blitz plan. And yogurt
made with live cultures can be a positive help by reintroducing those
healthy gut bacteria they tell you about in the adverts. But avoid fruit
yogurts, which are full of sugar and not remotely 'live'. Look for a
natural one that promises lots of 'probiotics' on the label.

CALCIUM

Calcium is a very important mineral. Without it, our teeth would rot, our bones would weaken, our blood wouldn't clot, we'd get muscle cramps and spasms, women would have menstrual problems, and we'd all have trouble sleeping. What's more, when our calcium levels are low, we are more prone to putting on fat because our bodies go into survival mode. If you decide to cut back on dairy products long-term, you need to make sure you get plenty of calcium from other sources, such as fish canned with its bones (eat the bones), dried figs, soya milk, tofu and leafy green vegetables. But don't worry for now: there's plenty of calcium in your Beach Body Blitz menu plan.

Changes to make

- What should you do if you take milk in your tea and coffee? Ideally, you should switch to alternatives such as green or white tea, or herbal teas (see pages 104–105), but if you really must have them, try to drink them black (and sugarless). Soya milk, rice milk and other cows' milk substitutes tend to separate in hot drinks, but all major coffee-shop chains offer soya coffees. Choose a 'skinny' one to cut calories.

- Instead of butter, choose an olive-oil spread for your bread. You avoid the lactose problem and have good fats instead of bad ones (for more, see page 101).

After the holiday is over, you can reintroduce dairy products if you wish, but take it gently. Try a sliver of hard cheese, such as Cheddar, first. Add a little milk to your tea, and wait a few hours to see if you react. Don't do this at the same time as you are reintroducing wheat, though, or you won't know which one is causing the symptoms.

Chances are, you may well be able to guess which foods are problem foods for you. What do you get cravings for? A bowl of pasta? A bar of chocolate? Or a double cheeseburger? Maybe your grandma used to say 'A little of what you fancy does you good' – but she was wrong. Often it's exactly the foods we crave that are causing us to bloat and put on weight, so bear that in mind next time the urge strikes.

Culprit no. 4 = red meat

Steak, chops, burgers and kebabs are all very difficult to digest. Heavens, they're even difficult to chew, so how's your poor old gut supposed to cope? If you eat a lot of red meat, chances are you've got undigested chunks of it tucked into crevices in your lower intestine, where they fester and give you that 'bunged up' feeling. We're not suggesting you have colonic irrigation, but if you did you might well see some of the remnants of a burger you ate years ago floating out amongst the other waste.

The Beach Body Blitz is designed to get your digestive system running smoothly and efficiently, so during the plan we don't want to clog it up with any more meat.

Red meat is high in calories and high in saturated fat – the bad kind of fat, the stuff that furs up your arteries and makes you more likely to have a heart attack. Just look at the comparative calorie and fat content of different kinds of protein (see the box opposite). It's pretty dramatic.

PROTEIN COMPARISONS, PER 100 G (3½ OZ) SERVING

	KCAL	FAT
LAMB CUTLETS, grilled	367	29.9
STREAKY BACON, grilled	337	26.9
PORK SAUSAGES, fried	308	23.9
PORK BELLY, grilled	320	23.4
ROAST BEEF	244	12.5
SALMON STEAK, grilled	215	13.1
ROAST TURKEY	166	4.6
CHICKEN BREAST, grilled	148	2.2
TUNA, canned in brine	99	0.6
COD STEAK, grilled	95	1.3
TOFU, steamed	73	4.2

The good, the bad and the ugly

What do nutritionists mean when they talk about good fats and bad fats? We need some fats in our diet to help us absorb vitamins and burn the calories supplied by proteins and carbs. But saturated fats, which are mainly from animal sources, have no useful function and when you eat a lot of them, your body simply transports it to your fat cells. That means your belly, hips and thighs. Hydrogenated fats, or trans fats, found in processed foods such as margarines and biscuits, are particularly bad for us and have been linked with several kinds of cancer as well as heart disease. These are the 'ugly' ones – but you can avoid them if you read the labels on packaged food carefully.

The good fats are monounsaturated ones, found in olive oil, nuts and avocados, omega-3 essential fats, found in oily fish, and omega-6 essential fats, found in pumpkin, sunflower, sesame and corn oil. These fats all have positive effects in the body, helping to reduce the build-up of fatty plaque in the arteries, lowering blood pressure and stabilizing blood sugar. Good fats have the same calories per gram as bad fats but because the body finds them useful they are not dumped so quickly in the fat cells to make us porky.

In fact, it seems that good fats are very helpful when you are on a weight-loss programme. People who eat oily fish in particular seem to lose weight much more rapidly than those who don't. You'll find plenty of salmon and tuna in the Beach Body Blitz eating plan, but when you are choosing your own meals again, you can get the same benefits from mackerel, sardines, herring, trout and pilchards. If you absolutely can't stand fish and nothing whatsoever will change your mind, take a daily capsule containing omega-3 and omega -6 oils. It's one of the most important things you can do for your health.

When you get back from your holiday, you can start eating meat again by all means, but opt for lean cuts and chop off any visible fat. It makes sense on so many levels – for weight control, for a happy gut, and for good health, too.

Culprit no. 5 = booze

Don't worry – we're not suggesting you give up alcohol for life. The Beach Body Blitz is only two weeks long. If you can't manage to stay booze-free for 14 days, it sounds as though you have a drink problem and you may need help to address it. We're serious!

Alcohol is not an essential for life. It's full of calories and it puts your liver under strain as it has to filter out all those toxic substances from the blood. By giving the booze a rest for a couple of weeks, your system will have a chance to clear out and replenish itself, leaving you feeling a hundred times healthier.

Here are a few of the reasons why we've made the Beach Body Blitz alcohol-free:

- Calories from alcohol are stored as abdominal fat. It's not called a beer belly for nothing, but it's not just beer that does it. Wine, whisky, gin, vodka, tequila – whatever your tipple, the calories will end up in a booze belly. Give yours a poke whenever you feel tempted to lift a glass.

- Booze is responsible for 'moobs' – man boobs – because when men drink too much of it their bodies are flooded with oestrogen, the female hormone.

- Drinking alcohol with meals makes us feel less satisfied by the meal and more likely to snack afterwards.

- After drinking a lot, we are drawn to high-fat, high-carb foods in an attempt to stave off the inevitable hangover, or to sugary foods in a vain attempt to fix those fluctuating blood sugar levels.

- Alcohol weakens your willpower, making you more likely to be tempted to over-eat.

- There are 187 kcal in a pint of bitter, 155 kcal in a double gin and tonic and 130 kcal in a large glass of red wine, but research suggests that they could make you fatter than a piece of cake with the same number of calories, because of the way alcohol calories are treated by the body.

- Excess alcohol is bad for your brain, heart, liver, gall bladder, pancreas, digestive system and kidneys!

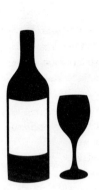

Enough said? When you follow *The Biggest Loser: Permanent Weight-Loss Programme*, you have the option of an alcoholic drink a day as part of your 'treats' allowance. You don't need to be teetotal to be slim. In fact, allowing yourself a treat after a day of good eating behaviour is psychologically important.

But, on the Beach Body Blitz plan, your treat is the forthcoming holiday and the vastly improved way you will look on the beach. Hold that thought.

Culprit no. 6 = fizzy drinks

Those little bubbles in beer, cola, ginger ale, bitter lemon, cream soda, lemonade, fizzy energy drinks and tonic water are bubbles of gas. And when you swallow them, the gas ends up in your stomach. If you are lucky, you will burp most of it back up again (lovely!) but it's more likely that a lot of it will end up further down your digestive system, where it will cause bloating and flatulence.

Over the years, dieters have often turned to low-calorie diet drinks, such as diet colas, but they are sabotaging their own efforts when they do so. Not only are they gulping down air, but they are also consuming artificial sweeteners that cause the insulin levels in the blood to rise and stop the body burning fat (see page 94). Amazingly, fizzy water drinks with a hint of fruit flavour fall into the same category. You'd think the combination of water and fruit must be good, and all the labels with poppy fields on a summer's day look gloriously healthy – but basically they are just sugar and gas.

Even plain fizzy water is a bad idea when you are thinking beachwear. We're trying to squeeze the gassiness out of your gut, not introduce more.

So what can you drink?

Water is the best drink option for cleansing your system. If you like you can add a few cubes of ice and a slice of lemon or lime. Keep some close at hand throughout the day and have a slurp whenever you fancy. It's important not to get dehydrated, especially when you are doing a lot of exercise.

All kinds of herbal teas are encouraged on the Beach Body Blitz plan. Some of them will positively help your detox efforts:

- Peppermint tea is good for the digestion. Get fresh mint leaves if you can and steep them in boiling water.

- Nettle tea cleanses the liver and is diuretic (meaning it makes you urinate more). This is useful for anyone prone to water retention.

- Choose tea blends containing milk thistle. Lots of companies make their own brand, which may be labelled 'cleansing tea'. It's good at helping the liver to shift toxins.

- Chamomile tea helps you to sleep well and it can also help to cure mild headaches.

How about coffee?

If this were a classic 'detox diet', we'd be telling you to avoid all drinks containing caffeine. That means coffee, tea (apart from herbal teas), cola and hot chocolate. Caffeine is a toxin that has to be filtered out of the blood by the liver. It can prevent nutrients we need being absorbed by the digestive system, and it tends to make cellulite worse (see page 193). Basically, coffee is a drug and if you normally drink five or more cups a day, you will probably get some withdrawal symptoms when you stop drinking it, such as headaches and difficulty concentrating. But we don't want to do that to you on the Beach Body Blitz!

It's definitely worth counting the number of cups of coffee you drink per day, and trying to cut down if there are more than three. Switching to tea instead would be a big help.

The average cup of filter coffee has 110 mg caffeine in it, while a cup of tea averages around 30 mg.

WHITE TEA AND GREEN TEA

If you haven't tried these types of tea, you could be pleasantly surprised by the delicate taste. They contain caffeine but are not harsh and have a pleasant-enough flavour to be drunk without milk or sugar. Both of them have huge benefits when it comes to health and, in particular, weight loss because they contain powerful substances that help the body to burn any fat in the bloodstream and prevent it being stored in fat cells. What's more, when you exercise they make the body release stored fat so that it can be burned – reducing your lumpy, bumpy bits and meaning that you are able to carry on exercising for longer.

If you've ever looked longingly at a packet of 'diet pills' in a chemist's shop or on the Internet, you can bet 'green tea extract' was one of the key ingredients. We don't recommend these pills because they tend to contain other substances that aren't so good for you. Why not get the green and white tea effect direct from a tea bag and benefit from this secret weapon that lots of thin people already know about?

Fruit juice

Fresh fruit juice doesn't contain as much fibre as the whole fruit, and the vitamin content deteriorates from the moment the fruit is cut open and squeezed, but it's basically a healthy drink. However, a large 300 ml (½ pint) glass of unsweetened orange juice can contain 108 kcal – which is a lot when your daily limit is 1,500 or 1,750 kcal. Apple juice could be even more – about 140 kcal. The sweeter the drink, the higher the calorie count is likely to be.

Fruit juices also give a blood sugar boost that triggers insulin to be released, so all in all it's best to avoid them on the Beach Body Blitz. Smoothies (see page 90) are fine as a healthy snack because the yogurt in them slows the uptake of the sugar.

After the two weeks are over, by all means drink fresh, unsweetened fruit juice again, but don't guzzle it back thinking there will be no calorie consequences. Because there are.

You can do it!

As you've found out, this two-week eating plan requires you temporarily to give up several foods that may be your favourites: bread, beer and burgers, chocolate and chips.

But it's only for two weeks (or four at most)!

Cheat if you want to. Keep drinking wine and dipping biccies in your coffee. It's no skin off our noses. The only person it affects is you. You're the one who's about to strip off on a beach somewhere. You'll be the one feeling self-conscious on the sand.

All we can say to you is that if you follow the eating and exercise plan exactly, you will definitely see substantial differences by the end of the two weeks.

- You will get rid of bloating and water retention.

- You will be less flatulent.

- Your digestive system should be working smoothly, without constipation or diarrhoea.

- Your skin will be clearer and eyes brighter.

- You will have improved muscle tone.

- You will shed weight and lose centimetres (or inches) in those all-important places.

- You should be sleeping well and feeling more energetic.

- You will definitely look much better in your swimwear.

Don't even think about the future at this stage. We'll talk about that later. For now, all you have to do is follow the plan to the letter and you will get results.

When you write about progress in your notebook every day, note down anything you have found especially difficult. Pat yourself on the back if you were sorely tempted to take a chocolate from a box that was being passed round at work and managed to resist. Write it down. That's a result! Keep your 'before' photos close at hand and have a private peek to remind yourself what you will look like on holiday if you give in to temptation.

Above all, keep a vision in your head of you stepping out onto the sand. Look at the travel brochure or search the Internet for pictures so you can visualize that beach clearly. Decide the colour of swimwear you would like to be wearing. Imagine yourself standing tall as you saunter down to dip a toe in the water. You might not be the perfect weight for your height but you will feel good in yourself, and you will enjoy your holiday. Go on – you can do it!

Choose some mantras and repeat them throughout the day to keep you motivated. Examples might be:

- **This year, I am going to have a fantastic holiday because I will be happy with the way I look on the beach.**

- **Every day I am getting slimmer, stronger and healthier.**

- **I will have a flat stomach on the beach.**

- **I deserve a great body, and I'm going to make sure I get one.**

Use these, or make up your own variations and write them in your Beach Body Blitz notebook. If you're alone, you can say them out loud, but otherwise repeat them in your head – and believe them, because they're true. If you follow our eating and exercise plans for two weeks, we guarantee you will be happier in your own skin.

CHAPTER THREE

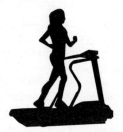

The exercise plan

If you are tempted to follow the Beach Body Blitz eating plan but leave out the exercise plan, think again. It's the exercises that will make the most difference to your appearance on the sand.

Here are a few reasons why:

- Shedding a bit of weight simply by eating less can leave you looking as loose-skinned and flabby as a jellyfish stranded by the tide.
- Even if you can't reach your ideal weight in two weeks, toned muscle creates a kind of optical illusion, making you appear trimmer and slimmer than you really are.
- Exercise burns calories. Exercising as well as eating less will more than double the effectiveness of any weight-loss plan. And with only two weeks to go, you need every trick in the book.
- How many dieters complain that they can never lose weight from the places they want to lose it? If you don't exercise, this is almost certainly going to be the case. Exercise will sculpt your figure, so that you lose flab from those embarrassingly wobbly bits.

- Once you build more muscle, your metabolic rate will increase so that you burn more calories throughout the day, even when you are just sitting on an aeroplane flicking through the in-flight entertainment options or travelling on a train to work.
- We won't bore you with all the health benefits of exercise, but suffice to say that if you are obese, you are in a high-risk category for dying prematurely. Regular exercise will lower that risk and help put you back into a healthy category.

At the end of the day it's up to you, though. Do your own thing. It's you who picked up this book because you weren't feeling confident about appearing in swimwear on a beach. Do you have the guts to do something about it or are you just an armchair reader? The world is about to find out.

You can disguise flabby bits in clothes to an extent but when you appear in swimwear, people are going to be able to tell at a glance if you work out.

The Beach Body Blitz exercise plan is not a stroll in the park. It requires a commitment from you of both time and energy. You'll need to set aside an hour before work in the morning, and almost an hour in the evening as well (although you can do the evening routine in front of the TV if you wish). No matter how much enthusiasm you have at the start, there are bound to be days when you can't be bothered. The trick is to just do it anyway. Don't give yourself the option. Treat it like showering, or doing the dishes after a meal. It has to be done for you to get the results you want. And it's not for long – it's only two weeks at the end of the day!

In fact, you will see and feel results pretty quickly – certainly by the end of the first week. Your morning sessions are designed to promote the release of serotonin, the happy hormone. After completing them, you'll feel a buzz and start the day energized and ready for anything. During the evening toning sessions, you'll be able to feel your muscles getting stronger day by day. By the second week, the movements will seem easier than they did before. And by the time you set foot on the sand, we guarantee that you will feel better in your own skin. You can't fail to if you follow the plan to the letter.

The natural girdle

Do you ever wear tummy control undies, such as magic knickers and body-shaper tights for women, or shapewear vests for men? These can help to flatten your flab under clothes but obviously you couldn't wear them on a beach without looking mighty silly. There's an alternative, though, and that is to strengthen your abdominal muscles to create a natural kind of built-in girdle. The exercises on the next couple of pages will do just this, and if you work hard enough you will see them starting to take effect within two weeks.

Flattening your stomach is not the only benefit of these exercises, though. You need to learn to brace your abdominal muscles properly in order to hold the correct position during all other kinds of exercise.

Strong abdominals protect your spine during movement and anchor you so that you are not pulled into awkward positions.

Lots of the exercises in the Beach Body Blitz workout will ask you to 'brace your abdominals' before starting, so you need to learn how to do it effectively.

Start by standing in front of a full-length mirror in your underwear. Let your stomach hang out. No, really let it all go. Don't worry – no one's watching! Now pull it in.

Most people who are out of condition will pull in the area round the belly button, creating a kind of scooped effect, but they probably won't be able to pull in all the muscles running between the bottom of the ribs and the pelvis. There's the rectus abdominus that runs vertically from the pubic bone to the breast bone; the transverse abdominals, which run across the area between the ribs and the pelvis; and the obliques, which tuck around the sides and give us a trimmer waist when they are toned.

You need to practise to get control of all these little critters – and here are a few things to try:

✗ Pull it up

The trick is to do this one without letting your back arch, so it is the abdominal muscles doing the work.

1 Kneel on all fours on a rug or exercise mat, with your hands flat on the floor directly beneath your shoulders and your knees positioned slightly apart.

2 Without moving your spine, breathe in and let your belly flop down towards the floor. Let it hang out.

3 Breathe out and use all your abdominal muscles to pull your belly back up, from your pelvic floor to the muscles just inside your hip bones and up to your ribs.

4 Let the flab flop out again and repeat 9 more times.

NEUTRAL SPINE

There are four natural curves in your spine: inwards at the neck and waist level and outwards at the chest and pelvis level. During exercise, you should aim to maintain these curves so that your spine stays in its natural alignment. Don't let your back arch as you move, and don't try to flatten your spine onto the floor when you are lying down. This is what it means when an exercise instruction says 'neutral spine'. Keep it naturally curvy and you'll keep it safe!

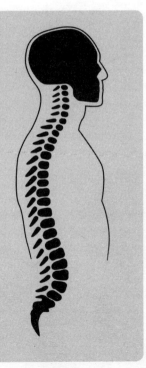

✗ Pull it down

This exercise helps you to feel all the muscles you need to get using. Pull down firmly as though you are trying to flatten your belly into the floor.

1 Lie on your back, with your knees bent and feet flat on the floor, roughly hip-width apart. Rest your fingers on either side of your lower abdomen, just inside your hip bones.

2 Breathe in, letting the breath push your fingers upwards.

3 Breathe out and use your muscles to pull your abdomen back towards the floor. Try to feel the muscles working under your fingertips. Repeat 9 more times.

✗ Pull it up and in

By working sideways, you strengthen the oblique muscles that will help to define your waist.

1 Lie on your side with your knees bent. Place a small cushion under your head and another one between your knees.

2 Breathe in and let your belly flop down to the floor.

3 As you breathe out, pull your belly up from the floor and then back towards your spine, in a kind of L-shaped movement. Repeat 9 more times.

✗ Pull it back

This is the hardest movement of all to control, but it's also the most useful because you can practise it virtually any time, any place: sitting at your desk, standing in a queue at the supermarket, waiting in the car at traffic lights or watching TV in the evening.

1 Either standing or sitting up straight, with a neutral spine, breathe in and let your belly hang out.

2 Breathe out and use all your abdominal muscles to pull your belly inwards and upwards, flattening the whole area instead of just scooping in the belly button. Hold for a few seconds.

YOUR PELVIC FLOOR

Both men and women should do pelvic floor exercises. They help prevent incontinence and impotence as you age, but they can also help you to strengthen your abdominal muscles. As you brace your abdominals, tighten the muscles between your legs as well and that will help to engage the muscles of the wider abdominal area.

Can't find your pelvic floor muscles? Sit in a chair with your knees slightly apart and feet on the floor, and lean forwards a little from the hips. Squeeze the muscles round your anus (both sexes), vagina (women), the base of the penis (men), then the urethra (both sexes – as if you are trying to stop urination). Hold for 10 seconds then release. The more repetitions you do, the stronger these muscles will get. (PS This is also good for your sex life.)

3 Repeat all day long whenever you remember. The more you do it, the stronger your muscles will get and the flatter your stomach will be on the beach. Simple!

The Beach Body Blitz Resistance Workout (see pages 136–185) will be working your abdominal muscles a lot harder than this, and it will be far more effective if you have good basic control over them.

Learning to pull your abdomen flatter is a wonderful skill that you will find particularly useful as you get up from your sun lounger to saunter down to the water for a cooling dip. Just keep holding it in until you are submerged in the turquoise waves. Then relax.

Warm up and cool down

You'll almost certainly have to get up earlier in the morning to fit in your first Beach Body Blitz exercise session of the day. It will take an hour all in, including 10 minutes of warm-up stretches, 45 minutes of fat-burning activity and 5 minutes of cooling down. Don't be tempted to skip the warm-up and cool-down because injuries are more likely to happen when you put pressure on tight joints and muscles. Stretched muscles and mobilized joints will resist stresses and strains, allowing you to do your workout safely and get the most benefit from it.

✖ Back stretch

You can do the first stretch of the day before you even get out of bed, to loosen up any stiffness in your lower back.

1 Lie on your back. Bend your left knee up towards your chest and catch hold of it with your left hand then repeat and do the same with your right knee.

2 Use your hands to pull the left knee closer in to your chest, then the right, then both together.

3 Keeping your hands on your knees, circle them round as if you are drawing a circle on a blackboard directly above you. Circle 5 times in one direction, then 5 times in the other.

Warming up

Now you're ready to get up and start the day! It's best to have your breakfast before doing the morning exercise session because you might get dizzy on an empty tummy, but leave showering until afterwards because if you do it right, you are going to get very sweaty! Pull on your exercise clothing, go to wherever you are going to be working out and get ready to do the rest of your warm-up, moving from top to toe.

✈ Neck stretches

Be gentle with these, and keep your spine neutral and your abdomen lightly braced throughout.

1 Standing straight, put your right hand over your head so it rests behind your left ear. Turn your head so you are looking towards your right armpit, holding your left arm down by your side. Gently pull on your head with your right hand, so that you feel the stretch in the left side of your neck. Hold for a few seconds.

2 Repeat with your left hand behind your right ear, pulling on your head until you feel the stretch in the right side of your neck. Hold for a few seconds.

3 Put both hands at the back of your head, with your fingers just beneath the bony edge of your skull, and your elbows pointing out in front. Gently pull your head forwards but at the same time resist the pull so that you feel the stretch in the muscles at the back of your neck.

✈ Shoulder release

This will really get the blood flowing into the shoulder joints and ease out any tension.

1 Standing straight with your feet hip-width apart and knees slightly bent, hunch your shoulders right up to your ears then let them drop down again. Do this 5 times.

2 Roll your shoulders forwards 5 times, then roll them backwards 5 times. As you roll back, squeeze your shoulderblades together.

3 Brace your abdominals, then circle your right arm backwards over your shoulder as if you are swimming backstroke. As the right arm starts to come down your back, raise your left arm to start a circling movement. Circle both arms together 10 times.

4 Now pretend you are swimming front crawl. Raise your right arm alongside your head then bring it forwards and circle it round. As it reaches the bottom, raise your left arm and start circling it as well. Circle forwards 10 times.

✗ Hip rotation

This is like oiling the ball and socket joints in your hips to get them ready to move smoothly.

1 Stand with your feet hip-width apart and your knees slightly bent, place your hands on your hips.

2 Brace your abdominal muscles and slowly circle your hips to the right, back, round and forwards. Repeat 9 more times.

3 Now circle round to the left, making the circle as big as you can. Repeat 9 more times.

✗ Quad stretches

The quads are the big muscles at the front of the thighs that we use when running, jumping and doing all kinds of fat-burning exercise.

1 Stand up straight and shift your weight to your right leg as you bend your left leg up behind you and catch the toes of your left foot in your left hand. If you think you are going to fall over, hold onto something with your right hand to help you keep your balance. Pull your foot up behind you as far as you can until you can feel the stretch in the front of your thigh. Hold for 20 seconds.

2 Put your left foot down and pull your right foot back as far as you can and repeat.

✗ Calf stretches

Calf muscles need to be stretched before exercise to prevent cramp or injury. They take a lot of strain, especially when you are running or jumping. Here's a good method that you can use wherever you happen to be.

1 Stand straight and take a big stride forwards with your right foot. Push your left heel down into the floor and you'll feel the stretch in your left calf. Hold for a few seconds, or longer if you are feeling stiff.

2 Straighten up, then step forward with your left foot to stretch the right calf. Hold for a few seconds.

This should do it for your warm-up, although feel free to target any other specific areas that feel stiff.

Cooling down

For a cool-down after you finish exercising, you can repeat any of the warm-up stretches that you think you need to ease out particular muscles, and then do the following stretches. Take it gently, holding each stretch for at least 20 seconds. Cool-downs help to get your heart rate back to normal and let any extra adrenaline in the bloodstream disperse.

✱ Side stretch

Feel your ribs opening with this stretch. Hold your abdominals firmly throughout to prevent your back arching.

1 Stand with your feet just wider than hip-width apart and your knees slightly bent. Cross your left arm across your waist and curve your right arm above your head with your palm facing forwards.

2 Brace your abdominals and bend to the left, stretching your right hand over as far as it will go and feeling the stretch in your right side.

3 Repeat with your left arm above your head, bending to your right.

✱ Hamstring stretch

Hamstring stretches are very important after any exercise that involves running and jumping, because the hamstring muscles (running from your butt down to your knees at the back) can get tight when you've been using your quads a lot. Here's a stretch you can do anywhere.

1 Stand up straight and step forwards with your left leg, bringing your foot down to rest on your left heel. Bend your right knee and rest your hands on it. Keep your upper body in a straight line.

2 Keeping your left heel on the floor, point the toes up towards you and you'll feel a stretch in the back of the left thigh.

3 Repeat the stretch with your right leg.

✗ Shoulders/triceps stretch

Shoulders can get tight after swimming, rowing, tennis and any sports that involve the use of the arms. Follow this routine to ease them out.

1 Stand with your feet hip-width apart, knees bent and butt sticking out slightly. Clasp your hands in front of you, palms facing forwards.

2 Push into your hands, feeling the stretch between your shoulderblades. Hold for 20 seconds.

3 Wrap your arms around your upper body, with your right arm above your left, and stretch them in opposite directions as far as you can.

4 Hold the position from step 3 and use your left forearm to pull your right elbow in towards your body, so you feel a stretch in your right shoulder. Hold for 20 seconds.

5 Repeat step 3 with your left arm above your right.

6 Hold the position and use your right forearm to pull your left elbow in towards your body.

✗ Lower back stretch

This is basically the Muslim prayer position! It's great for stretching tight muscles in your lower back and hips.

1 Kneel on the floor with your knees together, then lean forwards and stretch your arms out on the floor in front of you with your palms face down.

2 Slide your hands forwards and lower your upper body until your forehead is resting on the floor. Relax and feel the stretch in your spine. Hold for 20 seconds.

3 Slide your hands a few inches over to the left so that you feel more of a stretch in your right hip. Hold for 20 seconds.

4 Slide your hands to the right to feel more of a stretch in your left hip. Hold for 20 seconds, then slowly get up, ready to get on with your day.

Why not take a look at The Biggest Loser Club website for more warm up and cool down stretches (www.biggestloserclub.co.uk).

Fat-burning exercise

There are two main types of exercise: the fat-burning kind, known as aerobic, and the muscle-strengthening kind, which is sometimes called resistance exercise.

- Aerobic exercises target the largest muscle groups of the body and make them work at a rate that raises your heart rate and gets you sweating and at least a bit out of breath. If you're doing it right, your body releases fat stores to provide energy for the exercise, and you burn them up. Therefore you get thinner.

- In resistance exercise your muscles are lifting or pushing against a weight of some kind, whether it's your body weight or separate hand-held weights, and this causes you to build extra muscle tissue. The great bonus of it is that the more muscle you have, the faster your metabolic rate even when you are sitting still – so the more calories you burn even in your sleep!

For the best effects, any exercise programme should combine both types – and that's what we'll be doing in the Beach Body Blitz. First of all, there's the morning aerobic session of your choice (and then you will follow on with the Resistance Workout (see pages 136–185) in the evening. We would recommend choosing at least two or three different aerobic ones so you don't get bored doing the same thing day in, day out, but if, for example, you live near a tennis club and just want to play tennis every morning, that's fine – so long as you play energetically instead of pootling around on the baseline and stopping for chats at the net (see page 128).

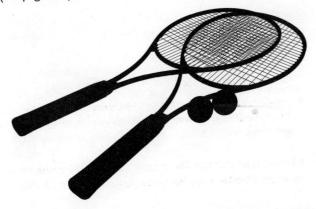

Choose what's best for you

Here's the list of choices, along with references to the page on which you will find more information about how to make it work for you. Tick at least two of them right now!

☐ Running/jogging/power walking (see page 120)
☐ Cycling (see page 122)
☐ Swimming (see page 123)
☐ Aquarobics classes (see page 123)
☐ Rowing/canoeing (see page 124)
☐ Skipping (see page 125)
☐ Rollerblading (see page 125)
☐ Trampolining (see page 126)
☐ Hula-hooping (see page 127)
☐ Ball sports, such as football and basketball (see page 127)
☐ Tennis (see page 128)
☐ Boxing (see page 128)
☐ Dancing (see page 129)
☐ Exercise DVDs (see page 129)
☐ Wii Fit (see page 130)
☐ Gym workout (see page 130)
☐ Aerobic classes at the gym (see page 132)
☐ Home workout (see page 132)

Your cardio options

Running/jogging/power walking

The only thing you need is a pair of running shoes – but don't think you can just slap on your mouldy old trainers. It's crucially important to get a pair of shoes that is right for the shape of your feet, your weight and the surface you are going to be running on. They need to fit well and be flexible enough to let your foot roll through from heel to toe, which trainers are unlikely to do. Visit a specialist running shop if you can, because the wrong footwear could make you injury prone.

Choose the route you run carefully. If there are uneven surfaces or objects in your path, you risk twists and sprains as you swerve to avoid them. A quiet park pathway is much better than a busy city pavement.

If you haven't run since you were a kid, don't launch straight into a full-blown sprint as soon as you get out the front door. After your warm-up, start walking and build up the pace gradually. Swing your arms by your sides, step out with your natural stride and walk as fast as you can without breaking into a jog. Keep this up for 45 minutes on Day 1, then do your cool-down exercises.

On Day 2, walk as fast as you can, but every now and then do a few minutes of jogging. On Day 3, you might be ready for 5 minutes of jogging and 5 minutes of sprinting in the midst of your power walking. Judge for yourself what you can manage. Don't overdo it, but remember that running burns the most calories of the three, so if you can work towards a position where you can manage the full 45 minutes at a mixture of running and jogging, you'll be shedding plenty of weight as you pound the pathway.

Wear a watch so you can time yourself, and see if you can beat your record from the last session each time. If you run with a Beach Body Blitz buddy, you can compete against each other – in a friendly, supportive fashion, of course.

RUNNING TECHNIQUE CHECKLIST

- Is your back straight and your back muscles relaxed?

- Are you looking straight ahead of you?

- Are you landing on the ball of your foot, with your toes pointing forwards? Heels shouldn't touch the ground.

- Think of the movement of your legs as being almost like cycling, with a circular motion at the hips. Thigh forward, leg stretched out, land on the ball of the foot when it is just below the hips, then push off.

- Try to avoid a lot of side-to-side movement at your waist.

- Keep your arms bent at 90 degrees, palms facing inwards, and let the arm movement come from your shoulders.

Cycling

Don't just borrow your kid's bike and expect it to work for an adult. There are specific rules for choosing a bike that is the right size for you and won't strain your shoulders, hips and knees or make you crash-land unexpectedly in a neighbour's front garden.

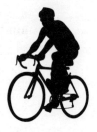

- When you stand over your bike, there should be a 2–8 cm (¾–3½ in) gap between the bar and your crotch.
- When you sit on the seat with your feet on the ground, your knees should be slightly bent (but not up round your ears).
- When you sit on the seat, hold the handlebars and put your feet on the pedals, roughly 40 percent of your weight should be over the bars, and the rest over the seat. Try to judge by the feel.
- Choose a bike with shock absorbers so you are not jolting your bones every time you hit a bump in the road.
- Wear a helmet to protect your head in the event of an accident.

If you are not an experienced cyclist it's a good idea to do a Safer Cycling Course before you start, to learn some tips on negotiating traffic. Most local cycling organizations or councils run something like this, and it could be a lifesaver. It would also be worth setting out early, before the morning rush hour traffic builds up.

Choose your route with care to avoid traffic jams and streets full of potholes. Select a circuit that is about 14.5 km (9 miles) long to start off with. This could be your route to work, so long as you are able to change out of sweaty clothes and have a wash when you get there. Most beginners should be able to attain an average speed of 19.3 km (12 miles) per hour over average terrain, so those 14.5 km (9 miles) should take you 45 minutes.

If you finish well within the 45 minutes, you can choose a longer route for the following session. More experienced cyclists can manage about 25.7 km (16 miles) per hour, so they should be able to manage 19.3 km (12 miles) in 45 minutes. Challenge yourself to keep it interesting – try and persuade someone to come with you to race against each other.

AQUAROBIC CLASSES

Working against the resistance of water increases the calorie burn.
If your local pool offers aquarobic classes, give them a try. If not, do
your own workout, as follows:

- Start with 10 minutes of jogging in water that is roughly waist depth.

- Follow up with 5 minutes of star jumps (see page 134 if you don't
  know what these are).

- Do a few minutes of squats (see page 140), pulling back into your butt
  and lifting your arms forward for balance.

- Stand on one leg and kick forwards then backwards with each leg in
  turn, holding your arms out for balance. Do this for 5 minutes.

- Crouch down so your shoulders are underwater. Extend your arms right
  out to the sides then bring them in to clap your hands. Do this with
  straight arms first, then bend your arms upwards at the elbows and
  bring them in and 'clap' your elbows together. Do this for 5 minutes.

- Lie on your front with your upper body on the edge of the pool and
  your legs just under the water. Paddle your legs up and down. Work
  really hard at this for 5 minutes and you'll feel your butt aching.

- Turn round so that you are sitting on the edge with your legs in the
  water. Place your hands flat by your sides for support and paddle your
  legs up and down for 5 minutes.

- Finish with 5 minutes more jogging round in the water.

Swimming

All you need is a costume, a towel – and a pool. Swimming is good
exercise for people who have weak joints because you are supported
by the water – but it is not a great fat burner, so don't choose this as
your only aerobic exercise. Do it twice a week at most, perhaps on
mornings when you feel stiff from a marathon session the day before.

If you haven't swum since school, consider taking a refresher lesson to
perfect your technique. You don't want to be one of those swimmers

who paddles along with your head held out of the water, trying not to get your hair wet. This causes the back to arch and will give you lower back strain. If you've forgotten how to breathe out underwater and then raise your head to breathe in, a quick class or two will remind you. You also risk injuring your shoulders with incorrect technique, so it's worth sorting out before you begin a fitness programme.

On the mornings when you choose to swim, put in lots of effort to get your heart rate up instead of pottering along in the slow lane. Alternate a length of front crawl, a length of back crawl, a length of butterfly, and only include the occasional length of breast stroke, because it's much more sedate and burns fewer calories.

One of the great benefits of swimming on the Beach Body Blitz plan is that you will get used to being seen in public in swimwear. Even if you scurry from the changing room and get underwater as quickly as you can, you've broken the ice and it will be a tiny bit easier when you disrobe on the beach in two weeks' time.

Rowing/canoeing

If you are lucky enough to live near a watersports centre, try rowing or canoeing for at least some of your morning aerobic sessions. Both are great exercises for anyone who wants to build muscle in their upper bodies, and they are good for the legs and abdomen as well. You need to brace your abdominals to anchor yourself on the seat as you push the oars or paddles through the water. You will use your legs to keep you steady in a canoe, and when rowing you'll need to use those big muscle groups in your legs to hold your position. If your only experience of rowing is on a rowing machine in the gym, you'll find it's much harder out on the water – but much more interesting.

Both rowing and paddling a canoe are great aerobic exercises if you approach them with gusto and you will see a difference in your muscle definition very soon after you start a regular programme. They are especially good for those with carrot shapes (see page 15), or guys who want to look a bit less weedy. If you get a chance to include either rowing or canoeing in your Beach Body Blitz exercise plan, grab it. Let's face it. With two weeks to go, fast results are what you need.

Skipping

You're unlikely to be able to skip non-stop for 45 minutes, but you could try 15 or 20 minutes and combine it with another aerobic activity to make up the time. Skipping is a high-energy, big-fat-burning workout that targets the shoulders, calves, thighs and butt, and all you need is a skipping rope and some soft-soled shoes that allow your foot to roll from heel to toe.

To choose the correct length of rope, stand on the middle of it and pull the handles up on either side. The point where the rope joins the handles should be level with your armpits. If it's not, tie knots in the rope to adjust it to the correct length.

Vary your workout by including some different skipping moves:

- Cross one foot behind the other, come back to centre then cross the other foot behind the other – turn about with each jump.
- Jump so that your left foot is forward and your right back, then switch for the next jump so your right is forward, and so on.
- Keeping your feet together, jump to one side and then the other.
- Jump your feet out wide, then back together, then wide again.
- Lift alternate knees up high as if you're doing an exaggerated kind of running step.
- Twist your upper and lower body in opposite directions, as if you are dancing the Twist.
- Change the direction of the rope and skip backwards.

If you have enough space, you can skip indoors in time to some energetic music. Aim for one jump every two seconds, 30 per minute. Wooden or carpeted floors are better than concrete because they have a slight amount of give and won't be so hard on your knees.

Rollerblading

As well as a pair of rollerblades, make sure you have protective clothing for when it all goes pear-shaped – as it will. The experts recommend a helmet, knee pads, elbow pads and wrist supports to cushion any falls. Don't let this put you off, though, because rollerblading is a very efficient calorie-burner and an ideal Beach Body Blitz exercise.

It can be a steep learning curve at the beginning as you learn how to keep your balance, push forwards, and stop as well. You start with your feet in a V shape, heels together, and push into each foot in turn, just as you would when ice skating. To stop, you use the rubber stop on the heel of one of your skates, touching it to the ground increasingly firmly and bending your back leg to give you greater control, almost as if you are sitting on the brake. If you fall (and you will!), try to fall forwards and land on your kneepads, then stretch your arms out to stop your head hitting the ground.

Once you've got the hang of rollerblading, glide off round the park, confident in the knowledge that not only do you look hip and trendy, but you are also going to burn several hundred calories in your 45-minute session.

Trampolining

You can buy mini-trampolines for the price of an Indian takeaway for two plus a six-pack of lager. One will get rid of your blubber and the other will add more. The choice is yours.

Trampolining is particularly good for toning up your waist, hips and thighs and the reason why we've included it as an option in Beach Body Blitz is that it could make your leg and butt muscles look more toned within the two weeks of the plan if you work hard.

Start off by doing small bounces in the middle of the trampoline (which is usually marked with a cross) until you are confident you have got the feel of it. Extend your arms and circle them to help you keep your balance. Once you're steady you can incorporate more moves to tone different areas:

- Run on the spot, pounding as hard as you can for as long as you can.
- Do some star jumps (see page 134) and each time clap your hands above your head.
- As you jump touch your right elbow to your left knee, then next time touch your left elbow to your right knee, and so on.
- Criss-cross your feet forwards and backwards and from side to side, alternating the foot that goes behind.
- Hop on one foot and then the other.

Invent your own variations, adding arm movements as well if you like. It's a fun but very effective type of aerobic exercise that you could do for your whole 45-minute session, or combine with something else, such as skipping – or hula-hooping.

Hula-hooping

Hula-hooping classes are springing up all over the place now. They're popular because it's not a difficult skill to master and the waist-trimming, abdomen-flattening results are well worth the effort. Don't pick up a kids' hoop from a toy shop, though. There are some adult stockists listed on page 223. To get the right size, measure the distance from halfway between your nipples and your belly button down to the floor – that is the circumference of hoop you need. If you have a particularly big waist for your height, add on a few centimetres (an inch). Bigger hoops are easier to use because they rotate more slowly.

To get started, stand inside the hoop and lift it up to waist level, holding it with both hands. Step one foot in front of the other. Push the hoop around your waist and shift your weight from your back to your front leg, trying to get the hoop to circle your waist without falling down. Don't circle your hips. Just rock back and forwards, shifting your weight from one foot to the other in the rhythm you need to keep the hoop in the air.

If at first you don't succeed, keep trying. With perseverance, you should have mastered it by the end of your first 45-minute hooping session, and you'll have burned off lots of calories along the way.

Tennis

It's a nice, summery, outdoor sport but your calorie burn during a tennis match will only be as good as the effort you put in. If you stand on the baseline knocking the ball back and forwards between you and your partner while keeping up a conversation, you're not working hard enough. A fast and competitive game with lots of running for wide balls and jumping for high ones is what you need to tone your arms and legs. Ideally, find an opponent who is at roughly the same level so you can challenge each other.

When choosing a racquet, it's always best to go to a specialist sports store to ensure you get the correct grip size. Go for a large-headed racquet and don't make the strings too tight so there's not too much vibration up your arm. It's definitely worth taking a few lessons to improve your technique and raise your game. Your tennis club is bound to have coaches who will give one-to-one sessions.

Keep up the momentum of the game, and collect your own balls between points. You should be out of breath after 10 minutes. If you are able to say 'That ball must have been in because it raised a cloud of chalk' without stopping for breath in the middle of the sentence, then you are not working hard enough.

Boxing

Most gyms now offer some form of box-ercise, kick-boxing or Thai boxing lessons as more and more of their members learn that it is one of the best all-over aerobic workouts you can do, with a huge calorie burn 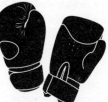 per session. You need to start with a class first to learn the basics, but you could then install your own punchbag from a rafter in a quiet area of your home and bash away at it! Alternatively, do some shadow boxing while holding hand weights (see page 135).

A classic boxing workout will include some skipping, squats and stretches as well as punching and kicking moves, and you will tone your arms, legs, chest, shoulders, waist, hips and butt. If there is a class locally, do consider trying it as one of your week's aerobic sessions at least. Don't worry – they don't actually punch each other.

Dancing

If you glanced down the list of aerobic exercises on page 120 and alighted on dancing as an easy option, then think again. Boogieing round your sitting room to your favourite music just won't cut it. Your 45-minute morning workout needs to raise your heart rate and make you sweaty and it's hard to sustain the right level of exertion when bopping away on your own. A high-impact aerobic dance class is the best option, and a quick Internet search should locate one in your area. Alternatively, try learning some 50s and 60s dance styles such as the Jitterbug, the Lindy Hop, the Twist or Swing dance. Salsa, tango and disco can also be fat-burning if done with conviction. Watch the movie *Dirty Dancing* for inspiration.

Belly-dancing has become increasingly popular recently, and if the midriff is your problem area then it could be ideal for you (although it would take a very brave man to attend a belly-dancing class). It's great for getting control of those tricky abdominals and training them so they are easier to flatten on the beach.

Exercise DVDs

The key is variety; plan ahead so that you are not doing the same thing day in, day out. We hate to blow our own trumpet but our Biggest Loser DVDs entitled 'The Biggest Loser Six Week Slimdown', 'The Biggest Loser New Year, New You' and 'The Biggest Loser Workout', offer a range of different workouts and some extras as well. It's a tough challenge, and will certainly get you burning flab from the word go.

If you want more DVD workouts to choose from, select ones with the words 'Burn', 'Ultimate', 'High Energy' or 'Challenge' in the titles and avoid any that call themselves 'Gentle' or 'Toning'. Some celebrity-led ones are good, while others are a bit wishy-washy (not naming any names). The programmes will probably incorporate their own warm-up and cool-down sections, but make sure the aerobic content in the middle lasts for 45 minutes. That's your Beach Body Blitz target, a key part of the overall plan that is going to give you a brand new body in just two weeks' time.

Discover how many calories you will burn by adding your workout to your online diary at The Biggest Loser Club (www.biggestloserclub.co.uk).

Wii Fit

Wii Fit takes the concept of exercise DVDs a bit further in that it can help you set personal weight-loss and fitness targets. Using sensors, it rates the intensity with which you are working and lets you know if you are slacking off. In fact, it's the next best thing to having a personal trainer watching over you.

You stand on a balance board, which will weigh you and can work out your body mass index (see pages 207–208) if you put in your height. You then choose your activity and, for the morning session, you should select aerobic ones such as running, a step workout, boxing or hula-hooping. Aim to progress to the more rigorous stages as fast as you can because some Wii Fit activities are a bit too gentle for our purposes. We have our own Biggest Loser game for Wii Fit, which we recommend highly!

One of the benefits of Wii Fit is that the steep initial cost should mean you keep using it, so as to get value from your investment. That console sitting beside the TV set should be enough to prick your conscience at least.

A gym workout

Joining a local gym is the best idea if you haven't exercised for a while, are over forty or have any joint problems, because you can work out in a supervised environment and ask for help if you need it. You will probably be given an introductory session by one of the trainers to familiarize you with the machines, and you can ask their advice on designing an aerobic workout that you can complete every morning in the run-up to your holiday. Make sure you know how to change the settings on the machines to suit your height, weight, leg length and the level of intensity at which you want to exercise. If they have heart rate monitors it's a good idea to use them so you know you are working hard enough to raise your heart rate, but don't let it get dangerously high.

Equipment that is suitable for your aerobic workout could include the following:

- All gyms have treadmills on which you can power walk, jog and run. Make sure you use a proper running technique, landing on the ball of the foot and pushing off the toes.

- Stationary cycles in gyms have a range of different settings so you can challenge yourself with hills and work at different effort levels. Push yourself until your quads and calf muscles are burning. Recumbent bikes, in which you lean back a bit, will target the abdominals as well.

- Stairmaster machines are fantastic for toning thighs and trimming the butt and you can set yourself challenges on some, such as climbing to the height of the Empire State Building (1,860 steps). Once again, you choose your effort level, and it can be really good to select a programme that combines easy and harder levels.

- On certain cross trainers you get a workout based on cross-country skiing. You hold onto poles and push your feet forwards as if trudging through snow. They target both upper and lower body, and once again it's the thighs where you'll feel it first.

- Rowing machines give you a great all-over workout, but you need to keep an eye on your posture to avoid strain. Keep your back straight and pull the bar directly towards your chest at nipple level. Don't let your knees drift outwards – they should stay in line with your feet throughout. Keep your abdominals braced to anchor you.

Your gym may have more aerobic machines, but you can get a really good workout with these five. Do 9 minutes on each, or do 15 minutes on three of them one day and another two the next. Mix it up to avoid boredom. And always remember to do your warm-up first and follow the session with a cool-down.

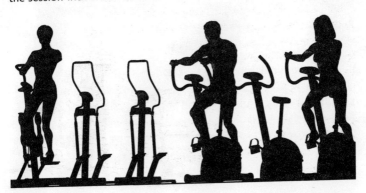

AEROBIC CLASSES AT THE GYM

You'll probably find a wide array of classes at your gym. Most of the
names should be self-explanatory but here are some terms you may not
have come across before:

- Spinning classes – these involve exercising on a stationary bike. Each
  person will have their own bike and a trainer will give instructions on
  whether you should stand or sit and which speeds you are aiming at.
  These tend to be tough classes.

- Step classes – you'll be given a plastic step and the exercises will involve
  stepping on and off it. Good for the hips and thighs.

- Circuit training – this is an exercise routine that works its way through
  all the main muscle groups of the body, using a mixture of aerobic and
  resistance exercises.

- Interval training – this mixes bursts of high-intensity exercise with
  periods of lower-intensity and works in a way that helps to increase
  your endurance, so you can manage to exercise for longer.

- Elliptical training – elliptical trainers are machines on which you can
  walk or run against resistance so you get a more intense workout than
  if you were simply walking or running normally.

- Martial arts training – lots of gyms offer classes that include elements
  of martial arts, such as kickboxing, t'ai chi and karate. These are all
  great calorie-burning workouts and definitely worth a try.

- Your gym may also offer yoga, Pilates, stretching and toning classes.
  These are all good for your body but they will not make you break a
  sweat so you can't count them as one of your daily aerobic workouts.

A home aerobic workout

If you can't get out of the house, perhaps because you have small
children to look after, then all is not lost. It's possible to give yourself
a good fat-burning workout without any DVDs, using just a few props.
Put some energetic music on the iPod that's around a beat per second
and work in time to it. Begin with your warm-up stretches, then do
each of the following exercises.

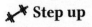 # Step up

If you can, get hold of a step designed for exercise. These will generally be about 90 cm (36 in) long, 35 cm (14 in) wide and around 20 cm (8 in) raised off the floor. If you can't get one, use the first step of your stairs instead.

1 Stand facing the step and bring your left foot up and onto the step, right foot up, left foot down, right foot down. Keep your back straight and your abdominals braced. Don't lean forwards into the step. Repeat 100 times.

2 Now stand with your right side to the step. Step with your right foot towards the back of the step then bring your left up alongside it. Bring the right down, crossing it behind the left, then bring the left down as well. Repeat 100 times.

3 Stand with your left side to the step and repeat step 2 bringing your left foot up first. Repeat 100 times.

4 Hold onto a banister or piece of furniture for support and stand with the balls of your feet on the step and your heels over the edge. Rise up on your toes then lower so that your heels are beneath the level of the step, feeling the stretch in your calf. Repeat 100 times.

Spotty dog

This exercise is named after the Dalmatian in a children's television programme. Aim to make yourself all floppy-limbed, just like a puppet on a string.

1 Stand straight with your arms by your sides to start. Jump your left foot forwards and right foot back, at the same time bringing your left arm up above head height and pushing your right arm backwards.

2 With a bouncing motion jump your left foot back and right foot forwards, left arm back and right forwards. Get into a regular rhythm of a beat per second and repeat 100 times.

3 Next do it with the opposite arms and legs in synch – left leg and right arm forwards, right leg and left arm back, then bounce to reverse. Repeat 100 times.

Star jumps

Also known as Jumping Jacks. We bet you can't manage 100!

1 Stand straight with your feet together and arms by your sides.

2 Jump your feet out wide and clap your hands above your head.

3 Jump your feet back together again and lower your arms. Repeat 100 times – or as many as you can.

Elbow to knee

This gives a nice rotation in the waist and a good leg workout.

1 Stand up straight and raise your left knee as high as you can, trying to touch it to your right elbow. You should be able to make them meet if there isn't too much blubber in the way.

2 Raise your right knee and try to touch it to your left elbow. Repeat 100 times with a good bouncing motion.

Side jacks

Keep working hard. Think of all those flabby fat calories you are burning with every repetition.

1 Stand with your feet wide apart and your hands held just in front of your breastbone, elbows bent outwards and palms down. Lean your weight into your right leg, keeping your spine neutral.

2 Jump into the air and when you land, transfer your weight to your left leg. Keep jumping from one side to the other, holding your arms up in front of your chest. Do 100 repetitions in time to the music.

Clean

Hold a hand weight for this – or a bottle of mineral water.

1 Stand with your legs just wider than hip-width apart, holding your weight in your right hand. Bow forwards, bending your knees and sticking out your butt so you are in a squat position. Keep your spine neutral and extend your left arm out to the side.

2 Bend your right arm to bring the weight up to shoulder height, at the same time straightening up and jumping into the air.

3 When you land come down into a squat again. Repeat 50 times with the weight in your right hand then switch to the left and do the same again.

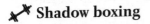 Shadow boxing

You'll need two hand weights for this exercise, which is great for strengthening the chest, arms and shoulders as well as giving you an aerobic workout.

1 Holding a weight in each hand, stand with your left leg in front of your right. Bring the weights up in front of your face with your palms facing downwards and elbows bent out to the sides, just like a boxer.

2 Punch straight out with your left hand, keeping your right hand close to your face.

3 Bring the left hand back and punch out with the right, feeling the twist in your abdomen. Repeat 100 times.

When you've finished, do your cool-down stretches (see pages 117–118) before collapsing in a heap on the sofa. We didn't say this was going to be easy, did we?

> *Minimum effort = minimum fat loss*
> *= maximum embarrassment on the beach –*
> *and the opposite is true as well.*

Once you've got over the initial exhaustion and had a shower, you should find that you feel energized. This amount of intense cardio will promote the release of serotonin, the feelgood brain chemical, and you'll face the day with renewed zing! Take any opportunity to keep up your activity levels during the day: stairs instead of elevator, walking to the shops instead of driving, using housework as an excuse for a bit of stretching and bending, keeping you nice and supple – all ready for your evening resistance exercise session.

The resistance workout

First, you need to get yourself ready. Eat your evening meal and do any chores that need to be done while the food is being digested, then get into loose, comfortable clothing ready for your evening session. This is the workout that is really going to hone your muscles so that the contours show through any layers of blubber. This is the one that will make you look fit rather than fat.

You will need:

- A rug or exercise mat
- A towel
- A couple of cushions

- Your resistance band
- Your dumbbells (see page 22)
- A 500 ml (17 fl oz) bottle of water

You can have the TV on in the background if you want so long as it doesn't distract you. You can't stop for 5 minutes to watch the screen or you'll lessen the effectiveness of the workout. It's better to work in time to some fast-paced, motivating music, of about 140 beats per minute. We want you to do these exercises FAST: boom, boom, boom, boom! You are aiming at 2 seconds for the first part of the movement, and 2 seconds to return to starting position. In the case of squats, for example, this will mean 2 seconds going down and 2 seconds coming back up again. Which is fast.

If you have any pre-existing joint problems or muscles weaknesses, seek advice from a medical professional before trying this or any other exercise programme.

This Resistance Workout is not for the faint-hearted or lily-livered – but it works. It will tone and sculpt all the main muscle groups of your legs, butt, back, chest, arms and abdomen, so that you look sleeker and fitter in your swimwear. And it will have ongoing effects as well, as your longer, stronger muscles will continue to burn extra calories long after the exercise session is over.

THE BURN

When you ask a muscle to perform hard work, such as lifting a weight, and there is not enough oxygen available as fuel, then your body creates its own fuel – a substance known as lactic acid – and burns it to keep your muscle working. In the old days, athletes used to be told that they had to hold back so as not to produce lactic acid, but now coaches and trainers recognize the value of forcing your muscles to work anaerobically (meaning 'without oxygen') because it improves their performance. Lactic acid means they can work stronger for longer. When you do your evening resistance workout, you want to feel that burning sensation in your muscles because that's what tells you that you are working hard enough. It should have gone again within an hour of stopping the exercise, as the lactic acid levels decrease.

Repetitions

To start with, you should do 10 repetitions of each exercise in the Resistance Workout (except where otherwise indicated). You should easily be able to manage this within an hour if you keep up the pace. That's more than a minute per exercise! Don't time every single exercise, but time yourself doing the whole workout from start to finish. The more reps you can manage without stopping for rests, the more toned your muscles will be.

- If you take longer than 1 hour to finish on the first day, you need to pull your finger out and speed up!

- If you take 1 hour or less, then on Day 2, you should try 15 reps of each exercise.

- Maybe on Day 3 you will get up to 20 reps. And who knows where you will be by Day 14?

On the first run-through, read the instructions carefully until you are confident you understand the movement. Remember all the advice on pages 110–113 about engaging your abdominals and keeping a neutral spine, because both are essential for protecting you from injury.

Putting in the leg work

You'll be working four major muscle groups in the legs: the quadriceps, hamstrings, adductors and abductors. These are all in the thighs, a place where many people have a tendency to lay down fat. Calves and ankles will get toned up without specific attention because they are indirectly used in every single exercise you do standing up, whether jumping, lungeing, squatting or stepping, but flabby thighs need all the extra help they can get.

The quadriceps (or quads) are big muscles at the fronts of the thighs that help you to straighten your legs. Are you sitting down as you read this? Put your hand on top of your right thigh, lift your right leg and straighten it. No matter how overweight you are, you should be able to feel your quad muscle doing the work in there. The quads are one of the body's powerhouse muscle groups, used in walking, running, cycling and almost all aerobic activities. The exercise plan on the Beach Body Blitz should give them a nice contour.

The hamstrings in the back of the thighs counterbalance the quads, and they are used when you bend your knees. To locate them, stand up and hold onto something for balance, then bend your right heel back towards your butt. You should feel the hamstrings pulling your lower leg back.

Adductors are muscles in your inner thighs that you use to move your legs inwards, while abductors are in the outer thighs and move your leg outwards. Stand holding onto the back of a chair, lift your right leg and move it across to the left then out to the right to get a feel for where these muscles are located.

In reality, none of these muscle groups work in isolation. When you use one, the others come into play to assist or counterbalance the movement. It's not as difficult to tone legs as it is for some other areas and you should be able to make a noticeable difference in two weeks. There will be no need to hide them under long trousers or skirts any more if you give these leg exercises all you've got.

✗ Leg extension

This exercise will start to fire up the quad muscles ready for their workout. If you don't have a resistance band, you can use a towel folded into a strip, but we strongly recommend that you get a band because they are such versatile, portable pieces of exercise kit.

1 Sit straight on a chair with your feet on the floor. Hold the ends of your resistance band or towel in both hands and loop it around the groove just in front of your left ankle. Lift your left foot off the floor and bring your hands back alongside your thighs.

2 Pull hard on the ends of the band or towel to provide resistance as you straighten your leg. Don't straighten completely or the band will slide up. Your quads will get plenty of work if you straighten by around 45 degrees.

3 Straighten your leg again and repeat 9 more times.

4 Switch and do the same thing with your right leg.

BUYING RESISTANCE BANDS

Most bands are colour-coded, with the darker colours indicating there is more tension in the band. It should also say on the packaging whether a band is more suitable for a beginner, or someone at intermediate or advanced level. If you are not particularly fit, why not buy a beginner's and an intermediate band so that you can challenge yourself by progressing once you have mastered the first? They're very reasonable in price and can be used in all sorts of ways in your exercise session. See page 223 for stockists.

✗ The basic squat

Squats are brilliant leg exercises, really making all the muscle groups do their stuff. There are lots of different variations, but in the first instance you should master the basic squat position and see how long you can hold it.

1 Stand straight with your feet hip-width apart, spine neutral and your abdominals engaged.

2 Bend your knees and push your hips back as if you are about to sit down on a chair. Aim for an angle of about 90 degrees at your hips. At the same time, lift your arms straight forwards at shoulder height, palms facing towards each other. Keep your head up and your eyes looking straight ahead. This is the basic squat position.

3 Hold the squat for as long as you can. Aim to manage at least 30 seconds the first time. You'll feel a burn in your thighs and butt, which means it is working and your muscles are getting stronger.

4 When you can't take any more, squeeze your butt muscles and use them to push you back up into a standing position again. Repeat 9 more times in quick succession.

Checklist:

- Have you kept the natural curves of a neutral spine, without increasing the arch of the lower back?

- Are your knees and feet pointing straight forwards, with heels directly behind your toes?

- Is your head up, eyes looking straight forwards?

- Are your arms roughly at shoulder height?

- Do you have a 90-degree angle at the hip? (Don't worry if you can't manage this at first, but resolve to work towards it.)

Now it's time to make that squat a little harder!

✈ The sumo squat (with dumbbells)

Have you ever seen sumo wrestling on the TV? These guys are huge, weighing 190–254 kg (30–40 stone) each. The biggest ever wrestler, nicknamed 'The Dump Truck', weighed in at 287 kg (just over 45 stone). But they are extremely fit all the same, due to a rigorous exercise and diet programme. Doing a squat in the typical sumo stance strengthens the legs in different areas, and holding a dumbbell will turn the intensity up a few more notches.

1 Pick up one of your dumbbells and hold it horizontal between the palms of your hands at chest height (just above the level of your nipples). Stand straight with your feet wider than shoulder-width apart with toes slightly turned outwards.

2 As you bend your knees to lower into the squat, keep your spine neutral and hold the dumbbell close in to your chest. Your knees should point in the direction of your toes.

3 Hold the position for 30 seconds and run through the checklist for the basic squat. Are you following all the points, apart from having your knees and feet turned out rather than straight?

4 Squeeze your butt muscles to come back up again, then squat down and come up 9 more times in quick succession.

✈ Dumbbell squat with knees

These squats are getting a bit more complicated each time, but all the basic rules still apply: neutral spine, abdominals engaged, head up and looking straight forwards. This time you'll need two dumbbells.

1 Stand with your legs hip-width apart, holding a dumbbell in each hand. Bend your elbows up so that the dumbbells are at shoulder height, with your palms facing inwards. Now lower into your squat. Yes, we know it aches by now!

2 Squeeze your butt muscles to come up out of the squat and, as you do, raise your right knee towards your left elbow. Award yourself a gold star if you can actually get them to touch.

3 Go back to the starting position and lower down into a squat again.

4 As you come up, raise your left knee towards your right elbow.

5 Repeat this 20 times – in other words, 10 times with right knee to left elbow and 10 times with left knee to right elbow. Work fast, allowing 2 seconds for each move. That means the whole exercise should only take you 40 seconds. If you can't get up to this speed straight away, resolve to work towards it as the two weeks progress.

✗ The ice skater

Think Torville and Dean or Dancing on Ice and glide smoothly through this exercise – which is another variation of our old friend, the squat. Put your dumbbells down, though. We don't want you dropping them on your toes. If you find you are very wobbly when you stand on one leg, it's something you should work at as it means your core muscles are not yet very strong. Practise whenever you can during the day.

1 Stand with your feet hip-width apart and spine neutral.

2 Drop down into a basic squat, then lift your left leg out behind you and balance on your right leg. It can help if you find a spot on the floor a few metres in front of you and focus on that. Let your arms relax by your sides.

3 Now jump up in the air and raise your arms straight out in front of you up to the level of your ears. It doesn't need to be an especially big jump but your foot should leave the ground.

4 Land on your left leg and bend your knee down into squat position, lowering your arms to your sides again. Check your spine is neutral and head is up.

5 Jump from leg to leg, bending as low as you can each time, then pushing upwards. Do it fast. Jump and land, jump and land, allowing 2 seconds for each move. That means that 10 repetitions on each leg should take you 40 seconds. Can you manage that? Brilliant! Pat yourself on the back.

🏋️ The kicking squat

Imagine the girls at the Moulin Rouge in Paris doing a can-can while holding dumbbells at the same time and you've got the gist of this exercise. Don't feel you've got to kick as high as they can manage though. Only go as high as you can reach comfortably.

1 Stand with your feet hip-width apart, holding a dumbbell in each hand. Let your arms hang by your sides, palms facing inward.

2 Go down into a squat, letting the dumbbells drop lower by your sides. Make sure your knees don't stick out beyond the level of your toes.

3 Squeeze your butt muscles, push out of the squat and kick your right foot up in the air as high as you can without losing your balance or straining anything.

4 Bring your right foot down and lower into the squat again.

5 This time, as you come up kick your left leg high in the air. Repeat 9 more times on each leg.

🏋️ The running squat

Before we finish with squats, we want you to try this high-intensity exercise, which is used by rugby players, sprinters and all kinds of athletes to intensify their muscle building. If you don't get the burn after this, you're just not trying hard enough.

1 Run on the spot as hard as you can for a fast count of 10. Really pound down into the floor.

2 After you reach the count of 10, drop down into a basic squat.

3 Squeeze your butt muscles to push up again and run on the spot for a count of 10. Repeat 9 more times.

✈ The jumping lunge

The lunge is another classic leg exercise, like the squat, with many different variations. Work through it slowly the first time, checking your position against the checklist below, before you speed up to the 2 seconds per movement we are aiming at in this workout. Once you have mastered it, you could hold a dumbbell in each hand, at hip level, palms facing inwards and elbows just slightly bent, to maximize the resistance workload.

1 Stand straight with your feet hip-width apart, abdominals engaged and a neutral spine, then take a big step forwards with your left foot. Keep your arms hanging loosely by your sides and your head up.

2 Bend your right knee down towards the floor so that your hips drop down. Your right heel will come off the ground and you'll take the weight on your toes. Lower yourself until you have a 90-degree angle at your left hip and left knee. Up to this point, this is the basic lunge position.

3 Jump up in the air and land with your right foot forward and left back in a reverse of the previous position. In other words, there should now be a 90-degree angle at your right knee and hip, while your left knee is bent down towards the floor. Keep the landing as gentle as you can; don't crash through the floorboards.

4 Repeat 9 more times each way, i.e. with your left knee forwards and right knee forwards.

If you are having trouble incorporating a jump into your lunge, just do a basic lunge to start off with. Follow steps 1 and 2 above, then push up through the front leg to raise yourself to starting position and repeat 9 more times each way.

Checklist:

- Are your abdominals engaged throughout?

- Is your spine neutral?

- Are both your feet pointing straight ahead and in line with your knees?

- Is your head up and eyes looking straight forward?

- Are you managing to get 90-degree angles at hip and knee? Try doing a lunge in front of a full-length mirror so you can check yourself from the side.

- As you jump, can you feel your leg muscles powering you upwards? Your butt muscles and hamstrings are activated in the front leg, and your quads and calf muscles are working in the back leg.

- Are you managing to land gently? Bending your knee on landing helps to absorb the impact so the action is not so hard on your joints.

✗ The tree

This is a yoga position that challenges your sense of balance and is especially good for the lower leg and ankle muscles. You'll find lots of different versions of this in yoga classes, where they try to balance with one foot right up at the top of their thigh in the groin. We've just given a basic version here to begin with, but feel free to slide that foot up further if you can.

1 Stand straight with your arms above your head, palms together.

2 Shift your weight onto your right leg and place your left foot on the inside of your right knee. Engage your abdominal muscles and hold for 10 seconds. You will undoubtedly be wobbling, but the adjustments you make to hold your balance as you wobble are strengthening those leg muscles.

3 Repeat standing with your right foot on the inside of your left knee and hold for 10 seconds.

Working your butt off!

Flat, saggy bottoms are sometimes cruelly labelled 'mum bums' but they are not exclusive to women who have given birth. In fact, they are a common complaint amongst people who spend a lot of time sitting on their butts. What do they expect? If you bought a nice plump cushion then sat on it for most of your waking hours, it would soon lose its shape. The exercises in this section are designed to make your rear more pert, so there's a bit more uplift and a bit less sag.

Another common complaint is 'saddle bags', where fat collects above your butt, to the sides, giving the kind of curves you definitely don't want on display. These are notoriously hard to shift but we'll do our best in the short time available!

It will be harder to make changes in the butt area than in the legs because if you don't exercise regularly, you're likely to have lost a lot of the muscle tone and laid down a lot of flab, but it should be possible to get it all looking a bit tighter within two weeks.

The main muscles giving shape to your butt are known as the glutes. They wrap around your buttocks and help us to make a range of different movements around the hip. Squeeze your buttocks together and you'll feel them working.

The hamstrings at the backs of the thighs also help to give shape to your butt, by lifting those saggy glutes, and the adductors that move your legs outwards are the ones that can get in and target the saddlebags. Are you ready to start working your butt off?

Side-lying leg lifts

Good position is essential for these leg lifts that target the adductor muscles, so be sure to run through the checklist below and correct yourself if you're out of line. You should feel a burn inside your butt cheeks as you work.

1 Lie on your left side with a cushion positioned under your head and a slim rolled-up towel under your waist to support your spine in its natural curves. Put your left arm straight up under the cushion, supporting your head, and rest your right hand on the top of your right thigh. Take a minute to make sure you are in a straight line. Now bend the left leg out in front of you to act as a stabilizer so that you can hold the position comfortably without falling over when you start to move.

2 Engage your abdominals and lift your right leg upwards, feeling the muscles working over your right hip. Only lift until your right foot is slightly higher than your hip. If you go any further, your waist will sink down and you won't be targeting the right muscles any more.

3 Lift up and down 9 more times.

4 Bring your right leg in front of you then up and back, making circles in the air, like a windmill. Get those circles as wide as you can without straining anything. Repeat 9 more times.

5 Now turn over and repeat steps 1 to 4 lying on your right side and raising your left leg. Repeat 10 times altogether.

Checklist:

- Are your shoulders directly on top of each other? And your hips? Don't let your trunk roll backwards or forwards during the movements – keep it straight.

- Is your spine supported in its natural curves?

- Can you feel the adductor muscles over your hip working as you move?

- Are your abdominals engaged throughout?

✈ The glute conditioner

This exercise has several parts to it, which should be followed in sequence. Each movement targets a slightly different area of your glutes. There's one that we refer to as The Peeing Dog; see if you can guess which one...

1 Kneel on all fours with your hands directly under your shoulders and knees under your hips. Engage your abdominals. It's important that you keep a neutral spine throughout this whole exercise and don't let your lower back sag downwards.

2 For the first part of the sequence, lift your left knee and bring it in towards your chest, then kick out backwards so your leg is in a straight line with your back. Repeat 9 more times.

3 Now bring your right knee in towards your chest and kick it out backwards in a straight line. Repeat 9 more times.

4 Go back to the starting position and extend your left leg out backwards so that it is in a straight line. Now bend your left knee at right angles so that your lower leg is pointing upwards and your thigh is parallel to the floor. Push your foot up towards the ceiling, then lower. Repeat 9 more times.

5 Repeat step 4 with your right leg extended backwards, pushing your right foot towards the ceiling.

6 Return to the position you were in at step 4, with your left leg extended out behind you and bent at the knee so your foot is towards the ceiling. Cross your left knee over behind your right knee and down towards the floor. Touch the floor if you can manage, then bring your left knee back up again. Repeat 9 more times.

7 Repeat step 6 with your right leg extended backwards, and crossing your right knee over behind your left.

8 Come back to the starting position on all fours. Lift your left leg and extend it outwards to the side. Try to get it as wide as you can. You won't manage an angle of 90 degrees to your body, but push towards this. Your leg should be straight and at hip height. Lift up slightly then bring it back in and down to starting position. Repeat 9 more times.

9 Do step 8 again, but this time lifting your right leg out to the side.

If you don't feel a burn in your buttocks, you're doing it wrong.
Go back to step 1 and work through the sequence again!

*Your back shouldn't move throughout the
Glute Conditioner sequence. You should be able to
lay a tray with a full cup of tea on it and not spill a drop!
(But it's not a good idea to try…)*

✗ The ski squat

You probably thought you'd seen the last of squats when you
got through the leg exercises, but this one targets the glutes very
efficiently. It's also useful if you're heading off on a skiing holiday
because it strengthens the muscles you use to hold yourself in a
skiing posture. It's just like a basic squat, but with your feet closer
together so it's targeting a different area.

1 Stand straight with your feet quite close together – just a small
   space between them. Engage your abdominals and check that your
   spine is neutral. Let your arms hang by your sides.

2 Drop down into a squat by bending your knees and sinking back into
   your hips, aiming for a 90-degree angle. Bring your arms forward at
   shoulder height, palms facing each other. Keep your head up and
   shoulders back.

3 Squeeze your glutes and press your palms together as you drive back
   up to the starting position. Repeat 9 more times.

THE MISSING CHAIR

Another good exercise for strengthening the glutes and quads is to
lean your back against a wall and shuffle your feet out roughly 30 cm
(12 in) in front of you. Slide down the wall until your hips and knees are
bent at 90 degrees, as if you are sitting down on a chair that isn't there.
Hold for as long as you can!

✕ The Bulgarian squat

This is called a Bulgarian squat because it originated in Bulgaria, home of those scarily big Olympic weightlifters and wrestlers. Remember that it's vital to maintain good posture when working with weights or you risk incurring some very nasty injuries, particularly to the spine. This will really push your hamstrings, glutes and quads to the limit, so get ready to burn, baby, burn.

1 Place a coffee table or low chair that's about knee-high a step away from you and stand with your back to it. Pick up a dumbbell in each hand and hold them by your outer thighs with your palms facing inwards, keeping your elbows very slightly bent. Lift your left foot backwards and rest your toes on the edge of the table or chair. Keep your right foot flat on the floor with the toes pointing forwards. Do a quick run-through. Spine neutral? Check. Abdominals engaged? Check. Head up and shoulders back? Check. OK, you're ready to go.

2 Keeping your back straight, slowly bend your right knee until it is at a 90-degree angle, or as close to that as you can manage.

3 Now drive hard into your right leg to push yourself back up to the starting position. Repeat 9 more times.

4 Change legs, so that the toes of your right foot are resting on the chair or table and you bend your left knee to lower yourself. Once again, repeat 10 times.

Muscles really burning? Give them a brisk rub before going on to the next exercise, but don't stop for a rest. You've got your metabolism all fired up now and your muscles are strengthening by the minute.

LET'S BE CHEEKY!

If the butt is a problem area for you, you can incorporate glute squeezes into your everyday life, along with pulling in your abdominals (see pages 110–113) and exercising your pelvic floors (see page 113). If you are subtle about it, no one need know what you're doing. You can squeeze those glutes while standing in a queue at the bank, waiting for your boss to read a contract, or even while chatting to someone on a bus. Just don't make funny, straining faces while you're doing it!

Here's a good standing glute squeeze routine:

1 Stand straight with your feet hip-width apart. Squeeze your butt cheeks together and hold for 4 seconds then release.

2 Squeeze the left cheek and hold for 4 seconds then release.

3 Squeeze the right cheek and hold for 4 seconds then release.

4 Squeeze both cheeks together again and rise up onto your toes while holding the squeeze, then come back down again.

5 Turn your toes outwards so you are making a kind of V shape with your feet. Squeeze your butt cheeks together and hold for 4 seconds then release.

6 Repeat over and over again.

You may find that one cheek is weaker than the other, in which case do extra squeezes on that side!

✈ One leg, one arm deadlift

The term deadlift sounds ominous. It's actually one of the disciplines involved in the Olympic weightlifting event, where contestants pick up a weight in a bent position and straighten as they lift it. In this exercise you'll do a single-handed deadlift. If you think it's hard, we would just like to point out that the world record for a one-handed deadlift is 330 kg (727 lb). How heavy is your weight again?

1　Stand with a stable chair or piece of furniture to your left side and rest your left hand on it. Hold a dumbbell in your right hand, just in front of your right thigh. Lift your right leg off the floor and out behind you so that you are balancing all your weight on your left leg. Take a moment to stabilize yourself. Make sure your spine is neutral and engage your abdominals.

2　Lean forwards, letting the weight of the dumbbell pull you downwards. Your right leg will rise up further behind you and your left leg will bend. Lean as far as you can while keeping your chin up and you will feel a stretch in your hamstrings.

3　Squeeze your glutes and push down through your left leg to bring yourself back up to standing position again. Repeat 9 more times.

4　Turn round so that the chair is on your right side and rest your right hand on it, holding the dumbbell in your left. Lift your left leg out behind you and repeat the exercise 10 times this way.

✈ Straight leg deadlift

Here's another deadlift, this time aimed fairly and squarely at those hamstrings that will tighten up the backs of your thighs and create an angle between them and your butt. It's like an anti-gravity lift, designed to fix the droop.

1　Stand with your feet hip-width apart. Hold a single dumbbell horizontally between both hands, so that it is just in front of your groin. Check that your spine is neutral and your abdominals engaged, shoulders down and head up.

2 Lean forwards letting the weight of the dumbbell pull you down, but this time keep your legs straight. You'll soon feel the pull on your hamstrings. Go as low as you can, hanging onto the dumbbell tightly so it doesn't drop on your toes.

3 Squeeze your glutes and push down into your heels to drive you back up to standing position again. Repeat 9 more times.

BUTT-LIFTING SHOES

Surely it's too good to be true? Some new ranges of shoes are available that increase the muscle activity in your legs and butt while you walk. They do this by introducing an element that wobbles in the sole, meaning you have to make constant little adjustments to stop yourself from falling over. The toes curve upwards and the shoes are weighted to encourage you to walk with good posture, placing your heel on the floor first and rolling through to the toes.

Many of us get into bad walking habits, especially if we are overweight. Have a look at an old pair of your shoes to see where they wore out first, and you'll be able to judge. If you get holes in the soles under the balls of the feet, you are leaning your weight forwards. Rundown heels mean you are leaning your weight backwards. Are you wearing out the insides or outsides? Is one shoe more worn than the other? All of these are signs that you are walking in an imbalanced way that will put stress on your knee and hip joints over time. Buying some of the new generation of shoes, boots or sandals will help to make sure you are balancing your weight squarely.

It can feel odd at first when you try walking in them, and you'll definitely feel a burn as your butt muscles begin to tone up. Want to try some? Go to http://uk.mbt.com or www.fitflop.com to find stockists near you.

Put your back into it!

Back fat is particularly unattractive fat. Women get rolls oozing over the top of their bra straps and squishing up into their armpits, men get flaps of it hanging down from their shoulderblades and both sexes get that unwanted extra roll curving over the top of their pants and joining up with the saddle bags at the sides. This is one good reason to do some exercises targeted specifically at the back area. The other is that strong back muscles protect your spine – and if you are overweight, your spine has more work to do than most. First of all, it has more weight to hold upright than the spines of slim folk. Secondly, your lower back is likely to be pulled out of position by your flabby gut, which can cause lower back pain, and women with big boobs are likely to get upper back pain as well as their spine strains to support the excess weight. Backache is the last thing you want on the beach, so read on…

The major muscles of the back are the trapezius, the rhomboids and the lats (or latissimus dorsi). The trapezius is a big diamond-shaped muscle at the top. Hunch your shoulders up to your ears and you'll feel it working. This is the one that can get bunched up and knotted if you've been poring over a hot computer for hours on end, or sitting tensed up at the steering wheel in the midst of gridlocked traffic. That's why we target the trapezius in the warm-up routine you do before starting an exercise session, with the Shoulder Release (see page 115).

The rhomboids are used to rotate your shoulderblades and pull them together. Try pulling them together right now and you'll feel where the muscles are.

The lats run from armpit level down to your pelvis and pull your shoulderblades downwards and your arms backwards. Try pulling your shoulderblades downwards and you'll feel them working.

There are other muscles involved, but these are the main ones we'll target in the back section. Ready to go? Get down on the floor then...

✖ Lower back raise

You may have come across this exercise before. It's something of a classic, and for good reason. You'll find versions of it in yoga, Pilates and all different kinds of exercise systems, but here we'll go for the straightforward method.

1 Lie on your front with your forehead resting on the floor. Bend your elbows at roughly 90 degrees and rest your arms on the floor with your palms down roughly level with the top of your head.

2 Engage your abdominals and slide your shoulderblades down your back, then lift your upper body off the floor. Lift your arms as well, keeping them in line with your upper body and head. Keep a straight line from the waist to the top of your head – don't bend your neck backwards. Hold for about 2 seconds, lower for 2 seconds, then repeat 9 more times.

CAUTION

If you suffer from recurrent back pain, don't ignore it in the hope that it will go away by itself. There could be any number of reasons: a torn muscle or ligament, one of the discs between the vertebrae in your spine bulging out, or wear and tear on the vertebrae causing pressure on the nerve. The sooner you get it treated, the less likely it is to deteriorate and cause long-term problems that could require an operation to correct. There are certain types of exercise you should avoid if you are prone to particular kinds of back pain, and only your health professional can advise you, based on the specific details of your case.

✖ Resistance rows

The movement you'll be making here is similar to that used in rowing and it works deep into the lats and rhomboids, as well as using muscles in your legs, forearms and biceps. Talk about killing several birds with one stone!

1   Stand on the middle of your resistance band, with your feet slightly wider than hip-width apart. Bend your knees and lean forward from the waist so that you can hold one end of the band in each hand, with your hands in between your knees, palms facing each other. Check that your spine is neutral. Pull your shoulders back and look straight ahead.

2   Engage your abdominals and pull your shoulderblades together then pull the ends of the resistance band up to waist level (or armpit level if you can). Keep your elbows close in to your body. Don't let them swing out wide.

3   Lower your arms to the starting position and repeat 9 more times.

✖ Reverse flies

All the back exercises in this section will improve your posture and, as we'll explain on pages 190–191, good posture can make all the difference in the world to the way you look in beachwear. Learning to hold your shoulders back does great things for your appearance, making women seem as though they've gone up a cup size and adding 7.5 cm (3 in) to the appearance of a man's chest.

1   Stand on the middle of your resistance band as you did for the last exercise. Bend forward at the hips, holding an end of the band in each hand. Your elbows should be slightly bent, and your hands just in front of your knees with the palms facing each other.

2   Engage your abdominals and lift your right arm out to the side and up to shoulder height. You'll feel the muscles working in the back of your shoulder.

3   Return to the starting position and repeat 9 more times.

4   You know what's coming next. Lift your left arm out to the side and up to shoulder height, and repeat this 9 more times as well.

*The level of difficulty of these exercises will be entirely
dependent on the tension in your resistance band.
If you are finding them very easy and aren't getting
a burn in your shoulders, buy a band with more tension
in it and do more repetitions.*

✗ Side bends

If we were to explain this to you in terms of the muscle groups and
movements, you might look blank, but when we say 'I'm a little teapot',
we're sure you will know what we mean. This exercise strengthens the
muscles of the whole trunk, not just the back. You'll find a version of it
in the cool-down exercises on page 117, but this one uses dumbbells
to increase the intensity.

1 Stand with your feet just a little wider than hip-width apart, holding
   a dumbbell in each hand, palms facing inwards.

2 Engage your abdominals and lift your right hand above your head.
   Hang onto the weight tightly!

3 Bend over to the left as far as you can, leading with your right hand
   and letting the left hand drop downwards to the outside of your left
   knee. Hold for 4 seconds.

4 Come back up, making sure your abdominals are firmly engaged and
   that your back isn't arching.

5 Raise your left hand over your head and bend to the left, then come
   back up to standing.

6 Repeat 4 more times in each direction.

✗ The pulley

We'll finish off the back section with some nice easy exercises you can do any time your shoulders feel a bit stiff or bunched up. For this one you need a banister strut or a sturdy handle of some kind that you can loop a towel around. Look round the house and we're sure you'll find something suitable. Choose a towel that is roughly a metre (yard) long and fold it lengthways a couple of times to make a band. (Don't try to use your resistance band for this or you'll fall over backwards.)

1 Loop your towel around the banister or handle and hold onto an end in each hand with your elbows bent by your sides. Stand with your feet shoulder-width apart just a few centimetres (inches) in front of the banister.

2 Engage your abdominals and lean backwards, keeping your feet in the same position and extending your arms. Go as far as you can without losing your balance.

3 Squeeze your shoulderblades together and pull yourself back up to the standing position. Repeat 4 more times.

✗ The push-off

This is good for engaging the lats, and it works the triceps in the backs of the upper arms as well – a notorious problem area that we'll be tackling later (see pages 172–173). Try it after a long day sitting at your computer to draw down the big trapezius muscles that tend to get bunched up.

1 Stand with your back against a wall, feet hip-width apart and a few centimetres (an inch) out from the wall. Hold your elbows by your waist and bend them so that your forearms are at right angles to your upper arms.

2 Engage your abdominals and push the backs of your arms into the wall so that your upper body comes forwards. Keep your trunk in line, and don't let your back arch.

3 Return to the starting position and repeat 4 more times. Easy, isn't it? Don't you wish they were all like this?

CHIN-UPS

Guys, if you want muscular shoulders and a strong upper back, there is no better exercise than doing chin-ups, which target the lats. You're unlikely to have a strong enough bar in your home, but all gyms have chin-up machines nowadays. You can use different grips to target different areas: palms facing you, palms facing away, further in or out. Be sure to start the movement in your shoulderblades, though, rather than trying to do the work with your biceps. These are great for girls as well, giving nice shapely shoulders. If you can't manage many full chin-ups, try one of the gym machines where you stand on a moving platform and choose the weight you want to pull up.

✗ The squeeze

This one uses a different set of muscles to draw your shoulderblades away from your spine, so it's good if you're feeling all knotted up. And it's another very easy one. Do more repetitions on the side that feels the tightest.

1 Sit on a chair or stool with your feet flat on the floor. Hold your elbows by your waist and bend them so that your forearms are at right angles to your upper arms. Slip a cushion between your left upper arm and your body.

2 Engage your abdominals and squeeze the cushion tight. Hold for 5 seconds and relax, then repeat 4 more times.

3 Put the cushion under your right arm and repeat the exercise.

Each of these exercises is trying to take the strain away from your shoulders and strengthen the muscles of the middle back. They are great for improving your posture and strengthening your spine.

Get it off your chest

Big boobs are supposed to be a good thing on a girl – but no one likes flabby boobs that wobble like a blancmange and plummet towards the floor as soon as her bra is unhooked. And boobs on a man are embarrassingly womanly, showing he has an excess of the female hormone oestrogen and a lack of underlying muscle tone. Firming up your chest needs a combined approach of eating less, cutting your booze intake and toning up the pectoralis major muscles (or pecs) that fan out from the breastbone on either side.

To feel your pecs working, put your right hand in your left armpit and lift your left arm into the air. Can you feel the muscle at work under the layers of flab? There is no muscle actually within your breasts – that's all fat and glands – but if you tone up the underlying pecs they will support breast tissue more successfully and help it to become more pert. The acid test, for men and women, is whether your nipples point outwards or downwards. If they're heading south, you'd better focus hard on the exercises in this section! And the first thing to master is the press-up.

The perfect press-up

Everyone, male or female, should learn to do perfect press-ups because they are the best chest exercise there is. We're going to do four different kinds in this section, each of them targeting a slightly different area of the pecs. Practise, practise, and more practise until you get them right.

1 Lie on your front with your hands on the floor beneath your shoulders and elbows tucked in to your sides. Curl your toes under. Check that your spine is neutral.

2 Engage your abdominals and push up so that your weight is just off the floor and resting on your hands and toes. Your body should be rigid, like a plank. In fact, we call this the 'plank position'.

3 Push down into your arms to raise yourself up until your arms are straight but the elbows aren't locked.

4 Keeping those abdominals engaged, bend your elbows and lower to the floor. Repeat 9 more times.

Can't do it? Not enough upper body strength? The only way to get stronger is to keep trying. Follow the advice in the box on page 163 if you can't lift yourself off the ground at all, but aim to progress as fast as you can to the full push-up.

Checklist:

- Are your hands directly under your shoulders? You'll make it harder for yourself if they are out wider.

- Are you dipping at the hips on the way up? You're doing it wrong then. Keep yourself in a straight line from heels to the top of the head, and that way you'll be able to harness your core strength.

- Are you keeping your elbows in as you push up? Don't let them stray out to the sides.

- Don't bend your head back or let it drop down. Maintain the natural curves of the spine.

- And keep those abdominals engaged all the way.

If you can't manage 10 press-ups, practise all night until you can. You won't be able to do the next five exercises without mastering press-up technique. Try, try and try again until you get there.

✗ Press-ups with a twist

This press-up variation uses more of the trunk muscles to trim your whole upper body. Try to rev the pace up. Can you do each step in 2 seconds? That would mean completing the 10 repetitions within a minute. Give it a try!

1 Get yourself into the basic plank position described in steps 1 and 2 of the Perfect Press-up (see pages 160–161).

2 Push up and raise yourself off the ground until your arms are straight.

3 Lift your left arm off the floor and turn so it is pointing straight up to the ceiling. Your weight will be entirely supported by the right arm.

4 Bring your left hand back to the floor and lower to the plank position again.

5 Push up and raise yourself off the ground again.

6 Lift your right arm and point it straight up towards the ceiling.

7 Lower to the floor again. Repeat 9 more times.

✗ Diamond press-ups

This works deeply into the pecs and enlists the triceps as well. Even though you perform it with bent knees, we think you'll still find it a tricky one.

1 Kneel on all fours and cross your ankles behind you. Bring your hands in beneath your breastbone, palms down, and make a diamond shape between your thumbs and index fingers. Rest your weight on your knees and hands, with your elbows straight but not 'locked'.

2 Keeping your elbows close in to your sides, lower yourself to the floor. Your upper body should stay in line from your knees to the top of your head. Touch your chin on the floor.

3 Push up again, with abdominals engaged and elbows close to your sides. Repeat 9 more times.

✕ Press-ups with applause

You'll have good reason to congratulate yourself if you manage to complete 10 repetitions of this dynamic press-up. Start by doing it on your knees, as described here, but when you get stronger you can try it pushing up from the plank position.

1 Get into the plank position (see page 161) and bend your knees, crossing your ankles behind you. Bring your hands out slightly wider than shoulder width. Check that your spine is neutral.

2 Engage your abdominals and push up hard, so that your hands come off the ground, with as much power as you can. Clap your hands together at the height of the jump.

3 Check your position on landing, then repeat. Try to manage 10 repetitions altogether.

FOR THOSE WHO REALLY CAN'T DO A PRESS-UP

1 Stand facing a wall, arm's length away from it. Place the palms of your hands on the wall just in front of your shoulders. Bring your feet together.

2 Keeping your back neutral, lean forwards until your nose just touches the wall and your elbows are bent in to your sides.

3 Now push into your hands to bring yourself back to starting position. Keep your elbows tucked in. Feel the muscles that are working. These are the ones you will need to do a press-up.

4 Now we're going to try the same thing, but with you in a horizontal position! Lie face down on the floor and place the palms of your hands under your shoulders. Bend your knees and hook your ankles together. Check that your spine is in neutral.

5 Push into your palms to straighten your arms, remembering to keep your elbows in by your sides. Even a five-year-old child can manage this! Focus on keeping your back aligned.

6 Lower again and repeat this as many times as you can. At your session the next day, try to do a full press-up again but if you can't, repeat this exercise 10 times.

Who says girls can't do press-ups? Keep trying and you'll make progress every day.

✈ The flying chest press

Lifting free weights is something you need to be taught how to do. If you walk into a gym, pick up the heaviest weights you can manage and attempt to lift them without proper technique, you will almost certainly injure yourself before long. It's important to keep a stable core so that the effort of the muscles as they lift the weight doesn't unbalance you and tear muscles. In this exercise, you have the floor to stabilize you so you shouldn't come to any harm. Unless you drop the weights, which you should try very hard not to do.

1 Lie on your back with your knees bent and feet flat on the floor, hip-width apart. Hold a weight in each hand. Rest your upper arms on the floor alongside your body, and bend your elbows so that your forearms are pointing upwards and your palms facing inwards.

2 Engage your abdominals and push your arms up straight so that the weights are directly above your shoulders.

3 Touch the weights together above your breastbone, bending your elbows slightly.

4 Open your arms outwards to lower the weights in an arc to the floor on either side of you, keeping the same slight bend in your elbows. You'll feel your chest opening up.

5 Bring the weights back up in the same arc shape and touch them together above your breastbone.

6 Bend your elbows and lower them to the floor by your sides so that you are back in starting position. Repeat 10 times altogether.

Do you have armpit fat that squidges out if you wear a sleeveless top? Toning up your pecs is the only way to target it.

✖ The burpee

We didn't make up this name – promise. It's a well-known, high-intensity body-conditioning routine that incorporates a few of the movements you've learned so far. This is an easy version. It can get much tougher, but we would rather you aim for speed in this workout. Can you do 10 repetitions in a minute? Top athletes can manage 30.

1 Stand with your feet hip-width apart and arms by your sides.

2 Jump into the air and as you come down lower yourself into a low squat position with your hands on the floor.

3 Crouch down on the floor, in a sprinter's start position then jump your feet back until you are in press-up position with straight arms.

4 Lower yourself to the floor then push up again.

5 Jump your feet forwards so you are in a crouch position with your hands on the floor.

6 Push up into a squat then stand up and jump in the air to finish. Repeat 9 more times.

Checklist:

Is this a dawdle for you? There are several ways to make it tougher.

- From the squat position (step 2 above), jump your feet back into press-up position. Then after you've done your press-up, jump your feet forwards into the squat.

- Want it even tougher still? Lower yourself into the press-up at the same time as kicking your feet back from the squat. Then push up again while jumping your feet forwards.

- Glutton for punishment? Why not go the whole hog and hold a pair of dumbbells while you're at it? Do your press-ups while leaning on them.

Up in arms

In summer, one glance at a person's bare arms is enough to judge whether they exercise or not. It's not difficult to get muscle definition in your forearms and upper arms, but if the only exercise you ever do is lifting a beer can or a jam doughnut to your mouth it will be obvious to any onlooker. You can spend the summer in long sleeves – or you can decide to do something about it. We're here to help.

The muscles we'll be targeting are the biceps, those Popeye muscles at the front of the upper arms; the triceps at the back of the upper arms, the ones that can tighten up your bingo wings; and the deltoids, which form the rounded curve of your shoulder. The forearm muscles will be exercised indirectly when you target the upper arms, which are more prone to flabbiness.

After the face, arms are more on view than any other body part. Wouldn't you prefer yours to be toned and attractive? Wouldn't you like to be able to wave at someone without your underarm swinging back and forth like a pendulum? You'll need your dumbbells throughout most of this section to speed up the process of turning that excess flesh into firm, honed limbs to be proud of.

Concentration curl

Do this slowly the first time, checking you've got the position and the movement exactly right. Then perform the rest of the 10 reps in 2 seconds each – up and down, on both sides. It's great for toning the biceps.

1 Sit on a chair with your knees bent and feet wide apart on the floor. Hold a dumbbell in your right hand and lean forwards a little so that it is hanging down between your legs and your right elbow is resting against the inside of your right thigh, just above the knee. Keep your head up and look straight ahead.

2 Bend your right elbow, curling the weight all the way up to your chest. Keep your wrist straight so the bicep does all the work.

3 Lower to starting position and repeat 9 more times.

4 Switch arms, holding the weight in your left hand and doing 10 fast repetitions.

If you don't have a sports shop near you, check out page 223 for stockists of dumbbells, resistance bands and other exercise equipment you can purchase online.

AVOIDING STRAIN

Have you ever watched someone in the gym trying to lift a weight that's too heavy for them? They'll go red in the face and the tendons in their necks will stand out with the strain. A dead giveaway is if they are holding their breath as they attempt the lift (which doesn't help, by the way). Follow this checklist to lift weights without tearing muscles and raising your blood pressure:

• Always warm up your muscles before lifting weights.

• Make sure the core muscles around your abdomen and pelvis are held firmly to stabilize you.

• As a general rule, breathe out as you lift and in as you lower.

• Use smooth, controlled movements. Don't jerk the weight up.

• Keep your wrists flat throughout.

• If you can't lift a weight slowly and smoothly, it's too heavy for you. Use a lighter dumbbell.

✗ Bicep curl and shoulder press sequence

There are several parts to this flowing sequence of arm-toning exercises, and you'll be doing 10 repetitions of each to start off with. Increase the reps if you can, and you'll see the differences in your arms even faster.

1 Stand with your feet hip-width apart, shoulders back and head up, holding a dumbbell in each hand with your arms by your sides and palms facing forwards. Stop to check your position: knees very slightly bent, feet pointing straight ahead, spine neutral, elbows by your sides, chin up, chest out. Ready to go?

2 Engage your abdominals and curl your arms up till your elbows are bent at 90 degrees and the weights are just below chest height. Keep your elbows close in to your sides.

3 Lower the weights to starting position and repeat this curl 9 more times. On your tenth curl up, keep your elbows bent at 90 degrees as this is the starting position for the next part of the exercise.

4 Bend your elbows further to bring your weights upwards and inwards to just above your shoulders. Keep your elbows tucked in to your sides throughout.

5 Lower to the halfway point with bent elbows again and repeat step 4, 9 more times. On the last repetition, bring your arms back down by your sides, palms facing forwards as in step 1.

6 Keeping your elbows tucked in, curl the weights all the way up in an arc from alongside your outer thighs up to your shoulders.

7 Repeat this curl 9 more times, but on the last one, keep your weights up above your shoulders, ready for the next move.

8 Open your elbows slightly so that your palms are facing inwards, towards each other. Breathe out as you push both arms up into the air directly above your shoulders. Don't stop until your arms are straight.

9 Lower the weights back to your shoulders again and repeat this move 9 more times.

You might think you don't need to engage your abdominals for an arm exercise but you risk injuring your back if you don't. Without a strong core, the movement of the weights could pull you off balance and tear the muscles supporting your spine.

ALTERNATIVE BICEP CURL AND SHOULDER PRESS

Resistance bands are convenient when you are away from home, as they are easy to pack into a briefcase or handbag. They are as effective at building muscle as dumbbells and the only disadvantage is that you don't know exactly how much weight you are lifting. Here's how to use them to exercise your biceps and shoulders.

1 Place one foot in the centre of your resistance band and hold the ends in your hands at hip level, palms facing outwards.

2 Engage your abdominals and slowly bend your elbows and curl the ends of the bands up to your shoulders. Keep your wrists straight and your spine neutral.

3 Repeat the bicep curl 9 more times.

4 Keeping the ends of the band by your shoulders, rotate your elbows upwards and outwards. Your palms should still be facing in towards your body. Push the ends of the band straight up over your head in a shoulder press.

5 Repeat the shoulder press 9 more times.

✗ The shoulder raise sequence

Keep your movements flowing and fast-paced throughout this sequence, which is slightly shorter than the last one – only slightly, though, and some of the moves are tougher. Keep thinking of the fact that it will make your shoulders look so nice, you'll want to take a big pair of scissors and hack the sleeves off all your t-shirts to show them off on your holiday.

1 Stand with your feet hip-width apart, knees slightly bent and arms by your sides. Hold a weight in each hand, palms facing backwards.

2 Engage your abdominals and raise the weights straight in front of you up to shoulder height. Your palms will be facing downwards.

3 Lower your weights to the starting position and repeat 9 more times, up and down, keeping your wrists flat and making your shoulder muscles do the work. Keep your spine neutral and your head up.

4 Stand with the weights by your sides, and turn your forearms so that your palms are facing inwards, towards your body.

5 Raise the weights straight out to the sides and up to shoulder height, with your palms now facing downwards. Keep your shoulders down, though – don't hunch them up. The weights should stay in line with your body – not in front of or behind it.

6 Re-engage your abdominals and bring the weights back down to your sides. Repeat 9 more times, watching your posture carefully. Keep that spine neutral!

7 Turn your forearms again so that the palms of your hands are now facing backwards.

8 Raise your weights in an arc, bringing your arms straight forwards and up above your shoulders.

9 Re-engage your abdominals and lower them to the starting position. Repeat 9 more times.

✗ Zip it up

The name of this exercise comes from the movement, which is like zipping up a coat or jacket. It's a good exercise for improving your posture if you normally have a tendency to slouch.

1 Stand with your feet hip-width apart, holding a weight in each hand just in front of your groin. Position them so that the ends of the weights are just touching and your palms are facing inwards, towards your body. Check your posture: spine neutral, shoulders back, head up.

2 Engage your abdominals, bend your knees and push out your butt to drop down into a squat position. The weights will now be in front of your mid thighs.

3 Jump up in the air and at the same time pull the weights up the front of your body as if zipping up a long jacket. Pull them right up to mid-chest height, keeping the ends touching and your palms facing backwards. Your elbows will be bent outwards in a V shape.

4 Lower the weights to the starting position and repeat 9 more times.

✗ Single-arm scarecrow

Imagine the way a scarecrow stands in a field forming a kind of cross shape due to the pole pushed horizontally through the sleeves of its old jacket. Except that the arms flop downwards where the sleeves are longer than the pole. If you can picture this, you've got the starting position for this great shoulder-strengthening exercise.

1 Stand with your feet hip-width apart and a weight in each hand. Extend your arms out to the sides in line with your shoulders then bend your elbows so that your forearms are pointing down towards the floor and your palms are facing backwards. Do the usual posture checks, including making sure your shoulders aren't hunched up.

2 Engage your abdominals and rotate your right forearm upwards, keeping the upper arm in line with your shoulder, until your palm is facing forwards. Your arms are now making a kind of swastika shape, with one forearm up and the other down.

3 Lower your right forearm again and repeat 9 more times.

4 Rotate your left forearm up and down in the same way, repeating 10 times altogether.

✈ Triceps chair double dip

Now we're going on to tone the all-important backs of the arms, which let so many people down. All three triceps exercises are simple to pick up; it's the repetitions that are the killer.

1 Sit on the edge of a chair with your knees bent and feet flat on the floor. Curl your fingers over the edge of the seat alongside your thighs. Now slide your bottom off the seat and shuffle your feet forwards so that you are resting most of your weight in your arms.

2 Lower yourself down until your elbows are bent at right angles, making sure your back stays straight and that you are looking straight ahead.

3 Push into your arms to lift yourself up to the starting position. Repeat 9 more times.

4 Now make it tougher. Straighten your legs so that you are resting on your heels. You'll feel this putting more weight into your arms. The triceps will have to work harder to raise and lower you now.

5 Lower down and push up again, aiming to get up to 10 repetitions. Give the backs of your arms a rub; they're bound to hurt after all that!

Tone your triceps by doing some chair dips during the working day whenever you find yourself with a spare moment. Always do at least ten at a time to get the burn that means it's working.

BINGO WINGS

Unfortunately, excess flesh in the underarms tends to be genetic and if your mum or dad had it, you'll have a tougher battle than most to firm it up. As well as all the triceps exercises, focus on your press-ups and try rowing, either on a lake or on a rowing machine in the gym. Some types of housework are useful: scrubbing the bottom of a pot is always a good one. And a final tip: scrub your arms with an exfoliant (see page 187) before you shower, to help break up the fat cells.

✖ The kickback

This one is a bit easier, and is useful because it targets a different area of the triceps. Check your position carefully to get maximum benefit.

1 Stand in the middle of a resistance band with your feet hip-width apart. Lean forwards so that your upper body is parallel to the floor and hold the ends of the bands with your palms facing backwards.

2 Push your left arm back as far as you can. Don't let any other part of your body move so that the triceps muscle is forced to do all the work.

3 Return to the starting position and repeat 9 more times.

4 Now push the right arm back and repeat 10 times altogether.

✖ The skullcrusher

This is yet another way to target those tricky triceps. Don't rush through this one though. Take it slowly and really feel the movements in the muscles.

1 Lie on your back with your knees bent and feet flat on the floor about hip-width apart. Hold a dumbbell in each hand and push them straight up in the air directly above your shoulders, with your palms facing each other.

2 Keeping your upper arms in the same position, bend your elbows and lower the weights back to rest alongside your ears.

3 Still without moving your upper arms, straighten your elbows and raise the weights up again. Basically, your elbows are acting like a hinge and your triceps are doing the work of straightening your arms. Keep your wrists flat and your chin up. Repeat 9 more times.

4 The next part of the exercise needs to be done one arm at a time. Still keeping your upper arms absolutely still, bend your right elbow and lower your weight diagonally across your upper chest to touch your left shoulder.

5 Straighten your right arm, and repeat this movement 9 more times.

6 Next, bend your left elbow and lower the weight to touch your right shoulder. Do this 9 more times and you're finished with triceps (and arms) for today!

Bust a gut

We've left the abdominal exercises to last, but in fact you've been targeting your gut all the way through, every time you engaged your abdominals. It all helps to bring the muscles under control, which will eventually flatten any overhang and re-create that waist you used to have way back in the distant past.

We've already talked about the three main muscle groups we'll be targeting, back in the section about creating a natural girdle (see page 110). There's the rectus abdominus, the transverse abdominals and the obliques. To get a better idea where they are, try the following:

- Sitting on a chair, press your fingertips into your stomach on either side of your belly button and lean forwards. Can you feel a muscle working in there? That's the rectus abdominus. Some abdominal exercises focus solely on this muscle but for a flat midriff you should target the other two main groups as well.

- Still sitting down, move your fingertips slightly away from the belly button on either side. Breathe out and pull your lower abdomen towards the back of the chair, as in the natural girdle exercises. The muscles doing the pulling back in this area are the transverse abdominals. Can you feel them?

- Now put your hands on your sides, just under your rib cage, with your thumb hooked round the back and fingers at the front. Keeping your hips on the chair, turn your upper body to the right and then to the left. Can you feel the oblique muscles working now?

No matter how huge your gut may be, and how much excess flab you need to shed, take heart from the fact that these big muscle groups are still functioning in there. All you need to do is strengthen them and make them do their job of holding you in more effectively.

✖ The perfect crunch

Now it's crunch time. If you've ever been to an exercise class before, you'll have done some version of crunches, but you might have called them 'sit-ups' or 'curl-ups' or some other name. Ours are tougher, and we'll be doing lots of variants so you need to perfect the technique to start off with.

1 Lie on your back with your knees bent and feet flat on the floor, about hip-width apart. Place your hands behind your head, elbows pointing outwards.

2 Engage your abdominals firmly, pulling them down towards the floor, then raise your upper body from the floor, leading with your breastbone. Keep your head up so that your eyes focus just beyond your knees. Hold for 4 seconds.

3 Re-engage your abdominals then curl a bit further up before lowering yourself slowly to the floor again. Do 10 repetitions, mentally ticking off all the points in the checklist below. Go slowly at first until you are sure you have got the movement right, then speed it up.

Checklist:

- Are your abdominal muscles engaged throughout? If your belly 'pops' up, you've lost control and need to re-engage.

- Are you leading the crunch with your head? This is wrong. Think of lifting from your breastbone, while keeping your neck in line with your spine.

- Is your chin up? Don't let it drop down into your chest. Imagine you are holding an orange under it.

- Don't try to curl too far. You're not trying to touch your forehead to your knees. It's more important to pull in those abdominals as deeply as you can and hold them tight.

- Keep your neck and shoulders relaxed. You shouldn't feel any strain in them.

Think you've got it? Now try some of the crunch variations (see pages 176–178).

✖ Roll downs

These are like a crunch done backwards, and they target the lower abdominals. They're good for people who need to strengthen weak stomach muscles. And if you're overweight, chances are that probably means you!

1   Sit up straight with your knees bent and feet flat on the floor. Extend your arms straight out in front of you with the palms facing down.

2   Engage the abdominal muscles then roll your upper body slowly backwards down to the floor. Use your abdominals to control the movement, which should be smooth, not jerky.

3   When you reach the floor, use your arms to push you back up to the starting position and repeat 9 more times.

WAIST-TO-HIP RATIO

Doctors sometimes use the waist-to-hip ratio (WHR) as a way of identifying patients with lots of abdominal fat, who will almost certainly have internal fat around their vital organs. This makes them at a much greater risk of heart disease, stroke and type 2 diabetes. You can check your own WHR by measuring your waist at the narrowest point and measuring your hips at the widest point. Then do the sum:

Waist ÷ Hips = WHR

A healthy WHR is below 1 in men and below 0.85 in women. However, you can have a decent WHR and still be too fat. Women with a waist measurement of more than 80 cm (32 in) and men over 94 cm (37 in) are considered to be at risk.

✈ The crunch twist

This one works the oblique muscles round the sides and is designed to give you your waist back again. It's in there somewhere, we promise!

1 Lie on your back in the basic crunch position, with knees bent and feet flat on the floor. Put your hands behind your head as before.

2 Engage your abdominals and lift your upper body off the floor, but twist as you lift, bringing your right elbow towards your left knee, and lifting your leg off the floor to meet it. See if you can make them touch in the middle.

3 Lower to the floor and as you lift bring your left elbow towards your right knee.

4 Lower to the floor. Do 10 fast repetitions of the whole exercise.

✈ Knees-up crunch

Targetting even deeper into the obliques, this will help to shrink any 'love handles' that would otherwise be bulging over the top of your swim shorts or bikini bottoms.

1 Lie on your back on the floor, lift your feet off the floor and bend your knees up in the air so that you have a 90-degree angle at both hips and knees. Place a water bottle between your knees.

2 Twist your legs over to your left side and bring them down onto the floor, with your knees at hip level and water bottle still held firmly between them. Keep your shoulders down on the floor. You'll feel a stretch in your right side. Now clasp your hands behind your head.

3 Engage your abdominals and lift your upper body off the floor, heading in a straight line towards your hips rather than twisting towards your knees.

4 Lower and repeat 9 more times.

5 Switch sides so that your legs are bent over to the floor on your right side, then do 10 crunches from that position.

Keep your abdominals firmly engaged when doing
crunches to avoid any strain on your spine.
Stop and re-engage if you need to.

✈ Reverse crunch

In this crunch, the movement is in the lower half of your body and you remain motionless from the chest up. It targets the lower abdominals, particularly little pockets of hard-to-shift post-pregnancy fat or 'booze bellies', where the calories from all those gin and tonics, beers and wines have been laid down.

1 Lie on your back with your knees bent and arms by your sides, palms facing down. Engage your abdominals and lift your legs straight up into the air, pressing down into your hands to help you balance.

2 Re-engage your abdominals and lift your hips off the floor, pushing your feet up towards the ceiling. Keep your legs straight. When you have gone as far as you can, hold for 4 seconds.

3 Slowly lower yourself to your starting position. You should feel it working deep within your lower abdominals. Repeat 9 more times.

PAIN

We want you to feel 'the burn' when exercising, but you need to distinguish between a burning sensation in the muscles that will dissipate within an hour after you stop, and the sharp pain of muscle tears or joint strains. If you feel any sharp pain, you should stop whatever you are doing immediately. Don't continue with any exercise that feels as if it is straining your back or neck. Stop exercising if you feel dizzy or sick. We push contestants on the Biggest Loser TV show to the limits, but that is done with the knowledge that we have a full medical team ready to step in. If you are exercising at home, you need to take responsibility for yourself. That brand new swimwear is not going to look so good when accessorized with a neck brace and elbow crutches.

⚒ Leg drops

These are tough. You need toned abdominals to do them. If you feel any hint of lower back pain, stop and go on to the next exercise, because it means that your abdominals aren't yet strong enough to manage this one.

1   Lie on your back with your arms extended out to the sides at right angles to your body and palms down. Raise your legs so that your feet are pointing straight up in the air. Don't lock your knees; there should be a slight bend in your legs.

2· Engage your abdominals and slowly lower your legs towards the floor. Push into your hands to help keep your balance. Go as low as you can without pulling on your lower back. You will probably be shaking with the effort.

3   Use your abdominals to pull your legs back up to starting position. Repeat 9 more times.

4   If you find you can manage Leg Drops without straining your lower back, congratulations! Why not try lowering your legs out to the side now? Hold your abdominals firmly, with your legs straight up in the air, feet together, and lower your legs to the floor by your left side.

5   Use your abdominal muscles to lift your legs and bring them over to the floor by your right side. Repeat 9 more times, but stop at any point if your lower back starts to arch off the floor or if you feel any discomfort in your back.

⚒ Leg shoots

Each of these abdominal exercises is targeting a slightly different area of the big muscle groups across your abdomen, so do them all in every workout. The more repetitions you do, the less wobble there will be in your belly as you trudge across the sand.

1   Sit on the floor with your knees bent and feet together. Put your hands on the floor behind you, fingers pointing away from you, and lean your upper body backwards so that it is at an angle of about 45 degrees.

2 Engage your abdominals and lift your feet off the floor, pushing into your arms to support yourself. Hold this position with your bent legs in the air for a couple of seconds to stablize yourself.

3 Shoot your legs out straight in the air, keeping your feet together and feeling the abdominal muscles controlling the movement.

4 Bring your feet back in, then repeat rapidly 9 more times without lowering your feet to the floor.

✈ Dead bug

You'll soon see why this exercise got its name because you're going to look like a beetle that has been turned on its back and is struggling to right itself.

1 Lie on your back with your knees bent and feet hip-width apart on the floor, and your arms straight up in the air. Engage your abdominals and raise your knees so that they are directly above your hips, and both your knees and hips are bent at 90 degrees.

2 Re-engage your abdominals then start the exercise. At the same time, straighten your right leg and lower it to the floor, while lowering your left arm to the floor alongside your head. Don't let your lower back arch at any point. If you feel it is going to, stop just before that point.

3 Pull your arm and leg back up to the starting position, then straighten your left leg and lower your right arm.

4 Repeat the whole exercise 9 more times, lowering the opposite arm and leg each time.

Each of these exercises targets a slightly different part of your belly bulge. If you can pinch more than an inch of abdominal fat, you need these.

✗ The Russian twist

The movement in this exercise, which originated in Russia, is like paddling a kayak, but you use your abdominals to centre yourself and stop you overbalancing. It's very effective for toning the obliques.

1 Sit up straight on the floor holding a dumbbell vertically in both hands just above your abdomen. Lean back a little, lifting your feet off the floor, and you'll feel your abdominals automatically engaging.

2 Twist your upper body round to the left and lower the dumbbell towards the floor on your left side, but without letting it touch.

3 Use your abdominals to reverse the movement and pull your upper body up and over to the right. Drive the dumbbell down towards the floor on your right side.

4 Pull up to the middle and repeat the whole exercise 9 more times.

✗ The plank

If you can remember 'plank position', which you learned in the section about press-ups (see page 161), then you are halfway there, but this version focuses on the abdominals rather than the chest muscles, and you rest on your forearms rather than your hands.

1 Get down on the floor with your legs straight and toes curled under. Bend your elbows directly below your shoulders and rest your palms face down on the floor. Lift your body so that your weight is supported on your toes and forearms. Is your spine neutral? If so, you will be looking down at the floor between your hands. Make sure your hips don't drop downwards.

2 Engage your abdominals and raise your left leg behind you so that your weight is balanced on the toes of your right foot and your forearms. You'll probably start to feel wobbly before long, but hold the position for as many seconds as you can. Keeping the abs strongly engaged is the key.

3 Lower your left leg and raise your right leg. Once again hold for as long as you can. Repeat 4 more times on each side.

✗ The commando

This starts from the same position as The Plank (see previous page) but it's a bit tougher. You'll find it in lots of army training regimes, if that doesn't sound too scary! We've included it here because it helps to build the abs, deltoids and pecs all at once.

1 Get yourself into the starting position for The Plank, with your weight resting on your forearms and toes and your abdominals engaged.

2 Shift your weight onto your right forearm and push up with your left arm until it is straight. Keep your body and legs in line, with your spine neutral.

3 Now push up with your right arm so that both arms are straight (but don't lock your elbows). Hold for 4 seconds.

4 Bend your left arm until the forearm is on the floor again. Do the same with the right arm. Repeat the whole exercise sequence 9 more times.

✗ Double leg lift

With the Side-lying Leg Lifts on page 147, you lay on your side and lifted the top leg. Here you are going to lift both legs from the same position. Sounds tricky? Give it a try!

1 Lie on your right side with a small rolled-up towel under your waist and a cushion under your head. Extend your right arm under your head and place the fingers of your left hand on the floor just in front of your chest, to help you keep your balance. Run down your body to make sure you are properly lined up: your shoulder joints should be directly on top of each other, hip, knee and ankle bones directly on top of each other, and your spine should be supported in its natural curves.

2 Engage your abdominals, stretch out both legs and, keeping them together, lift them off the floor. Just a small lift is best. Hold for 4 seconds then lower again. Repeat 4 more times.

3 Turn onto your left side, get into position and lift from that position. Repeat 4 more times.

WAYS TO KEEP ACTIVE THROUGHOUT THE DAY

• As you brush your teeth in the morning and evening, lower down into a Sumo Squat (see page 141) – but obviously without the dumbbells. Keep repeating throughout your teeth brushing session. (Note: don't try this while shaving or applying eye make-up though!)

• While getting dressed, don't sit down to pull on trousers, socks or tights. Balance on one leg so that you are using all your core muscles to stop you falling over. If your partner is watching, it'll give them a good laugh to start the day.

• While standing at the sink washing dishes or sitting behind the wheel of your car, alternate between abdominal pull-backs (see page 112), glute squeezes (see page 151) and pelvic floor exercises (see page 113).

• Think of a way to make your commute to work more of a calorie-burner. Get off the bus two stops early and walk; cycle or rollerblade; if you have to drive a car to work, park further away and walk back. If you work from home, hop, skip and jump down the hallway to your office.

• Keep moving during the day. Volunteer to be the one who goes to make tea for everyone else; take the stairs to the photocopier, even if it's on the 14th floor; stand up whenever you make a telephone call.

• Turn housework into an aerobic workout, squatting as you push the vacuum cleaner under the sideboard, doing Side Jacks (see page 134) as you dust, and performing some bicep curls (see page 168) as you pick things up off the floor.

• Have a radio playing in the background and every time a track you like comes on, get up and dance energetically.

• If you have a partner, give them a treat by getting more lively under the duvet. Tell them to lie back while you do all the work, and you'll reap the benefits in oh so many ways!

Feel the progress

We don't recommend that you weigh and measure yourself every 5 minutes on the Beach Body Blitz. Apart from anything else, there might be days when your weight goes up slightly as your body builds muscle tissue, and that could be disheartening. The aim of the exercise plan, as we've said before, is to tone, trim and make you look better on the beach. It's good for morale, though, if you can see progress as you go along, and that's why we suggest you try to increase your effort level every day.

- Compete against yourself (or a friend) in your chosen form of aerobic exercise: running or cycling further in a faster time, managing more lengths of the pool or more bounces on your trampoline. Keep a note of your achievements in your Beach Body Blitz notebook (see page 18) and give yourself a big tick whenever you break your previous record.

- In the evening Resistance Workout, try to increase the number of repetitions by five every day. It should be possible because the exercises will get easier as you become familiar with them and your body 'remembers' how they work. Note down how many repetitions you have managed at the end of each session.

- Note also if you have difficulty with any particular exercise. Don't give up on it unless it causes sharp pain (see page 178). Go back and try it again during each workout and gradually it should become easier as your muscles get stronger.

All the exercises will seem easier by the end of the first week because your body will have changed already, even if you can't yet see the difference.

By the end of week one, you'll notice that you have much better control over your abdominals, which is going to help you manage all the other exercises more smoothly. Your legs and arms will also get stronger reasonably quickly, because the muscles won't be quite as out of condition as those in your trunk: you've been using them every day, even if you never did any formal exercise sessions. Stubborn areas of fat, such as saddlebags, man boobs, love handles and bingo wings, won't disappear overnight, but they will gradually be tightening up as

GET REAL!

You shouldn't need any help to stay on the Beach Body Blitz plan for two weeks. It's only 14 days, for goodness sake! That's just 28 hours of exercise and 42 delicious low-calorie meals. Either decide you are going to pull out all the stops and commit to this plan wholeheartedly – or don't bother.

There's no point if you're not going to follow the eating and exercise plans exactly. If you start missing the odd morning session because you're 'feeling knackered', or cutting some exercises from the evening session because your favourite TV programme is coming on and you're not finished, you won't see the changes you want by Day 14. There's no room for days off, or 'treats' or slackening the pace. This is an all-or-nothing plan. End of story.

you do your 2 hours of exercise a day. You may feel clothes fastening a little more easily and you may not. That doesn't matter. What will matter is the way you look on Day 15 when you slip into your swimwear and walk out onto the sand.

Keep your goal in sight. Look at pictures of the beach resort you are going to. Read reviews of your hotel on the internet (see websites such as www.tripadvisor.com), which will tell you what other visitors thought of it. Picture yourself there, lying by the pool with a novel in your hand, or strolling along the edge of the ocean feeling the sun on your back and the sand between your toes. Now look at the 'before' pictures you took. That's not how you want to look on the beach, is it?

Stay focused on the reason why you picked up this book in the first place. In the next chapter we're going to look at more ways you can improve your appearance on the beach – and they don't involve exercise. Promise!

CHAPTER FOUR

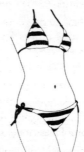

Looking great on the beach

Slowly but surely you are trimming down and shaping up ready for your beachwear debut. Meanwhile, we have several more suggestions for making you look your absolute best on the sand – and what's more, most of them aren't even painful!

It's a classic rule that to draw attention away from your worst features, you should maximize your assets. What are your best bits? Do you have great hair? A sexy décolletage? Stunning eyes? A lovely smile? People who have been overweight or obese for a while tend to have low self-esteem and some don't like any aspects of their appearance. If you can't think of a single bit of you that is attractive, ask a friend and we're sure they'll tell you straight away. Everyone has something going for them.

Once you've decided on your best assets, just go for it.

- **Get a haircut that flatters your face. As you slim down and the cheekbones re-emerge, a different cut might emphasize them. Tell the hairdresser you are going on holiday and need an easy-care style.**

- Both men and women can benefit from a spot of eyebrow shaping. Nothing too drastic or you'll look permanently startled, but neat, shapely eyebrows draw attention to the eyes.
- Do you wear glasses? Is it time to try contacts? Or change the shape of your glasses to suit the shape of your face better? Follow the advice on choosing sunglasses below.
- Have your teeth whitened. It's the single most effective way to make you look younger, and will enhance a gorgeous smile.
- Girls – go to a make-up counter and ask them to create a natural beach look for you, with a slick of highlighter on cheek and brow bones and a curl of waterproof mascara to open up your eyes.
- Have a manicure and a pedicure. Most people's feet are ugly after a winter shoved into boots and shoes. Get that hard skin filed off and your cuticles and nails shaped and you will have four more body parts you don't need to be embarrassed about on the sand.
- Exfoliate daily in the shower to get rid of the old layers of flaking, bumpy skin and expose a smooth new surface. Rub an exfoliator vigorously all over your body, then shower off.

SUNGLASSES

An attractive pair of sunnies that suits the shape of your face can the thing people first notice about you. To choose yours decide your face shape – round, oval, square or long.

- If you have a round face, avoid small, circular glasses and opt instead for rectangular lenses or cats'-eye shaped lenses that curve outwards at the upper edge.

- Those with oval faces can get away with most shapes. Choose wire-framed aviator ones, or try on the season's must-have fashion shape to see if they are flattering.

- Strong-boned square faces look best with thin frames surrounding round or oval lenses.

- Long faces can appear shorter if you wear frames with a pronounced bar across the top at eyebrow level. Avoid small square shapes.

Your holiday wardrobe

Two or three days before your departure date, go back to the department store where you did your 'before' shots (see page 18) to pick out the swimwear you will take with you on holiday. You may not have the perfect figure yet but you will look a darn sight better than you did when you took those candid shots in the changing room mirror. This time you are going to find some beachwear that will make you look good rather than emphasizing the flaws. Here's some advice on camouflaging techniques.

Remember – regardless of your body shape – don't squeeze into a smaller size than normal just to prove you can. If it digs in and makes you bulge over the top, you'll not be doing yourself any favours.

Beer guts

Guys, if your waist is still bigger than your hips, avoid tight Speedo-style trunks that will emphasize the overhang. Slightly baggy swim shorts or knee-length board shorts will balance your shape. Avoid neon. A big swirling pattern or a colourful check in dark will be most flattering.

Wobbly bellies

Girls, if your tummy wobbles when you laugh, you will probably want a one-piece swimsuit. The ones with tummy control panels can work wonders. A deep V-shape neckline will draw attention to your cleavage rather than your belly. A flowing pattern will be more flattering than a solid colour, but opt for darker shades. Alternatively, if your wobble is all in the lower abdomen, perhaps the aftermath of a pregnancy, then a tankini style could hold it in.

Big butts

Don't go for anything skimpy on the lower half. Bikini bottoms that are at least 7.5 cm (3 in) deep round the sides will work best. The ones with little skirts are good, but avoid any frills or flounces that draw attention to your butt area. Keep it plain down below and choose a top with some kind of decorative detail to lead the eye upwards.

No waist

If would like to appear more curvy, you could choose a one-piece that is cinched in at the waist, either with a belt or with tummy-control panels. If you've been working hard on the oblique muscles, try an all-in-one with cutaways at the sides, which will automatically give you curves. Alternatively, choose a bikini in which the bottom half ties at the sides, giving an optical illusion of width, and team with a padded top to balance it.

Huge bust

Underwired tops offer the best support and there's less chance of falling out of them. Halter necks are good for enhancing the cleavage, but make sure they have adjustable straps you can alter to fit properly. You'll feel more secure with wide shoulder straps rather than narrow spaghetti ones.

Short, stumpy legs

Choose a suit that is cut high on the thighs to lengthen your legs. A self-coloured bikini bottom paired with a fancier top will also help by drawing the eye upwards. Avoid any unusual styling in your bottom half that will attract attention towards your legs.

QUICK AND EASY BEACH COVER-UPS

Nipping to the beach bar for a refreshing drink? Slip a little something on top of your swimwear to cover up the bits you don't want to advertise. For women, the best option is often a sarong tied casually round the waist, covering the butt and backs of the thighs, but with a hint of leg showing through the opening at the front as you walk. If you're self-conscious about your top half as well, you can tie your sarong just above the bust, or pull on a short, loose kaftan (but not a full-length one – and don't wear the kaftan with the sarong). Men can throw on a baggy short-sleeved shirt and leave it open or just fasten a couple of buttons over any offending moobs or excess gut.

Posture power

Have a look at the adverts for slimming products that feature 'before' and 'after' shots and you'll often notice that at least half the reason why the 'after' shots look so much better is that the person is standing up straighter and taller. That's exactly what you're going to do on the beach from now on.

Once you've bought your new swimwear, bring it home and try it on in front of the mirror to assess your posture and look at ways you can improve it. The difference can be immense – and this is where all your girdle-bracing exercises will prove invaluable.

1 In bare feet and wearing your new swimwear, stand sideways on to the mirror without attempting to hold your stomach in.

2 Now pull in your abdominals as you've been practising and see how you appear instantly taller and straighter.

3 As you look at your side view, your shoulders, hips and knees should be in line with each other. If your shoulders have a tendency to hunch forwards, raise them up to your ears and let them drop back naturally to get into the correct position.

4 Now turn to face into the mirror. Still holding in your abdominals, try to lengthen the distance between your pelvis and your ribs. You might add as much as 2.5 cm (1 in) to your height when you do this. Pull your ribs upwards so your spine is stretched to its full extent, but without hunching your shoulders. Keep them relaxed, with your arms hanging loosely by your sides. This is the look you want.

The next thing is to learn to walk like this. Start practising walking with your abdominals braced and spine lengthened as you go around the house and out to the shops. Swing your legs loosely from the hips and try not to be too stiff. It should feel natural before long.

Remember that holding and lengthening those abdominals has a double function: it makes you look thinner, and all the time you are holding those muscles you are strengthening them.

Girls, those high heels look good but they aren't great for posture. They tilt the pelvis forwards, making your butt stick out, and you then have to arch your back and lean your upper body backwards for balance, pushing your bust out. By making you taller, heels can give the illusion that you are thinner, which is all for the good, but don't wear them for long periods or you could damage your back over time. Besides, you'll just look silly tottering along the sand in stilettos. Why not get some of the new generation of flip-flops (see page 153) with specially designed soles that give your legs and butt a workout as you walk? They really work, and they look great too.

Keep an awareness of your posture at all times. This doesn't mean marching around like a sergeant major, but it does mean holding your abdominals in slightly and keeping your spine neutral. You'll look better, and you'll be doing your back a favour as well. Keeping your shoulders back and down will make your chest look better, whether you are male or female. When sitting in a beach café with a cool drink and a light salad, sit up straight. Have a look at those celebrity beach photos we mentioned earlier and remember that slouching creates extra belly rolls.

TIPS FOR TOP BEACH PHOTOS

Even the skinniest bikini models will stand slightly sideways to the camera with one leg just in front of the other. There's a reason for this. By narrowing the appearance of your legs, it gives you a slimmer and curvier silhouette than if you were facing the camera squarely. Men will also find it more flattering to stand slightly side on to the camera. Keep your abdominals pulled in and your chin up to avoid the appearance of multiple chins. If you are being photographed sitting down, watch out for tummy wrinkles. And NEVER turn your back to the camera when you're in swimwear. Not ever. Not for anything.

Be your best self

After all the trouble you've taken to trim and tone your figure with the Beach Body Blitz, you might as well use all the other cosmetic short-cuts to looking good on the beach that are readily accessible and inexpensive. In for a penny, in for a pound.

Depilation decisions

One or two days before departure, it's time to think about depilation. More and more men are having unsightly areas of back hair removed and some decide to do their chest as well. All we can say is that it's a matter of taste, but it could be worthwhile if you look as though you are wearing a gorilla suit.

For girls, depilation generally means legs, armpits and bikini line. Try on that new swimsuit again to check whether your bikini line needs a tidy, then choose your method:

- Waxing, either at home or in a salon, should give you smooth, hair-free skin for the duration of a two-week holiday.
- Depilation creams are pain-free if a bit smelly, and they should see you through at least a week stubble-free.
- Shaving has to be done daily and you could have stubble appearing by evening.
- Electrolysis is permanent but it's expensive for larger areas and you'll need several sessions to catch all the hairs.

To fake or not to fake?

White wobbly bits look much worse than tanned wobbly bits, and you're going to attract unwanted attention if you resemble a giant snowdrift in the middle of the sand. A quick covering of fake tan could help you blend in with your surroundings and camouflage cellulite and other lumpy, bumpy bits as well.

If you've never tried faking it before, the day before your flight is not the best time to practise. Novices can end up looking like an orange tie-dyed 1970s sofa cover. Our advice? Splash out on a salon tan for the best results. They know what they're doing. You don't think those golden-skinned celebrities do it themselves, do you?

If you prefer to DIY, follow the golden rules: exfoliate first, apply moisturizer to rougher areas such as knees and elbows, spread the fake tanner all over and wash your hands immediately afterwards. Body lotions with a hint of fake tan are good, but you'll need to use them for several days before you see an appreciable result. It can also be helpful to buy products that tint the skin as you apply them, making it easy to see the bits you've missed.

THE TRUTH ABOUT CELLULITE

FACT NO. 1
About 95 percent of women have cellulite to some extent, but only around 5 percent of men. Its development is partly related to the female hormone oestrogen that makes women curvy on their hips and thighs. Fat cells under the skin become compressed, creating a dimpled, orange-peel effect that is much less prominent on men, partly because they have thicker skin.

FACT NO. 2
There are loads of different causes. Eating too much fat and sugar, drinking too much caffeine, yo-yo dieting, and certain vitamin and mineral deficiencies can all contribute. So can spending too much time sitting on your butt.

FACT NO. 3
There's not a lot that so-called 'miracle' creams or 'anti-cellulite tights' can achieve. A healthy diet and plenty of regular exercise can help to prevent cellulite forming, and some experts recommend regularly brushing affected areas with a stiff brush or massage glove to help break up the worst patches.

FACT NO. 4
Liposuction could actually make it worse, because the artificial removal of fat can create grooves and dimples under the skin, which are difficult to fill out again.

How do you measure up?

The evening before your departure, it's time to see how far you've come in your Beach Body Blitz journey. Strip down to your underwear and get out the tape measure. Take your chest, waist, midriff, hip, arm and thigh measurements in centimetres (or inches) and write them in the 'after' column in your notebook (see page 18). Don't be disappointed if you haven't reduced every single measurement. If you've replaced fat with muscle, you will look a whole lot better regardless of what the numbers say. Similarly, if you weigh yourself and haven't lost as much weight as you had hoped, it's probably because you've replaced fat with muscle, which is heavier. It's not what the scales say but how you look that counts.

Now put on your new swimwear and take the 'after' photos, remembering to follow all the postural advice on pages 190–191. Take a front, side and, if possible, back view. Print them out and compare them to your 'before' photos. Aren't you glad you Beach Body Blitzed it?

You may not yet have the body you want –
years of over-eating and under-exercising can't be
turned around in a fortnight – but you are bound to
look much better than you did two weeks ago.
Hold that stomach in and feel proud!

If you were working with a Beach Body Blitz buddy, call them and compare results. Be sure to congratulate them on their success, and thank them when they do the same for you.

Eat your final Day 14 meal, do your last exercise session and pull out your suitcase to pack for the holiday. Why not try on some old favourite outfits from the days before you let yourself get plump? You could be pleasantly surprised to find that they fit once more and look good on your newly toned frame.

As you try them on, check out the reflection in the mirror from different angles. It's important that you feel comfortable and relaxed in your clothes and aren't walking around worrying if your bum looks big or if a fitted top gives you 'bra sausages' at the back. Do as Kate Moss does and check yourself from every angle before you leave home. Ask a trusted friend to advise if that will help to build your confidence. Only pack outfits that make you feel good.

While packing, remember to include anything that will maximize your assets. A well-chosen necklace, a pretty hairgrip, or a shirt in a colour that brings out your eyes will mean that's where people look first. And after a good first impression, they'll be much more charitable in their subsequent summing up.

The main thing is that you take with you all the tools you'll need to relax and enjoy your holiday: the right clothes, deodorant, sun cream, talcum powder if you are prone to chafing, a sunhat to keep you cool, your sunglasses, and some great books. Now pick up your passport, tickets, money, phone… and get ready to relax!

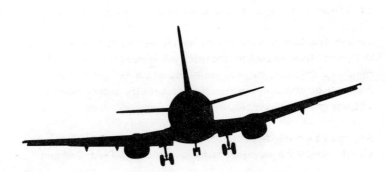

CHAPTER FIVE

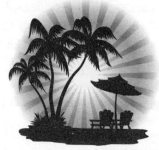

Enjoying your holiday

You'll be glad to hear that you don't have to take your Beach Body Blitz notebook on holiday with you. There's no strict eating or exercise plan to follow during your break, although there are certain tips you should stick to if you want to avoid undoing all that good work in one huge gluttonous binge. It might be a good idea to take your 'after' photos along to remind yourself that you actually look OK now and can feel proud of how far you've come. You are in control of your own body and your own health, and that's the way you can stay.

The number one rule when you step out onto the beach for the first time is to act confident. Nothing attracts unwanted attention more than someone with bad posture who is hunched over and skulking along trying not to be noticed. If you stand straight and walk tall, the truth is that most people will barely glance at you. They won't be whispering about your cellulite and giggling about your gut because they will notice your good posture and well-chosen swimwear, cool sunglasses or flattering haircut.

Most people are self-conscious on beaches,
worrying about their own paunches or stretch marks,
or the fact that they've just discovered their bikini
goes transparent when wet.

They will be spending far less time checking you out than you'd imagine – unless, of course, they fancy you.

Just a few things to watch out for:

- Check the position of your swimwear before emerging from the water, just to ensure nothing has slipped sideways, making you expose more than you would ideally choose to.
- Don't sit on woven lattice chairs with bare legs. Put down a towel. Nuff said.
- Keep applying the sunscreen, and don't overdo the sunbathing. On every beach that Brits visit, there's always at least one who is scorched to a painful shade of raspberry. It looks especially awful on flabby flesh – even worse than winter white.

Eating and drinking on holiday

You want to relax and enjoy your break without counting calories or weighing portions at every meal. It's very hard to stick to a rigid diet when you're not in your own kitchen, without subjecting waiters to a detailed inquisition about every single dish – and are your language skills up to that? At the same time, you want to keep your stomach unbloated and as flat as possible, so follow these three golden rules:

1 No wheat.
2 No cow's milk or cheese.
3 No fizzy drinks.

That shouldn't be too hard, should it?

By all means have an alcoholic drink or two, but avoid gassy ones like beer or you'll soon blow up like the Michelin man. Try a local cocktail with fruit juice, or a glass of wine with lots of ice clinking around in it.

Have a meat dish if you feel like it, but avoid the creamiest, fattiest options (see the list of suggestions for food choices in different countries that follows).

Regard ice cream sundaes and elaborate desserts with caution. They are the devil come to tempt you. Check out the calorie/exercise equivalents chart on pages 203–204 and when you are tempted to lift that spoon, think again.

These are the main rules and they should be easy to stick to no matter where you are holidaying, but here's some specific advice for some of the most popular destinations.

Britain

Choose: seafood, such as oysters, prawns, crab; all kinds of roast meat with boiled instead of roast potatoes and no gravy or sauce that's been thickened with flour; grilled fish, chicken or steaks; game, such as venison or partridge; kedgeree.

Refuse: bread, full English breakfasts, fish in batter, anything in pastry, sponge puddings.

China/Hong Kong

Choose: clear soup; steamed fish with ginger and spring onions; stir-fries with beef, chicken, prawns or vegetables; crispy duck (without pancakes); rice or rice noodles; Chinese vegetables, including beansprouts and water chestnuts; fresh lychees for dessert (but not the ones canned in syrup).

Refuse: dim sum, wontons, prawn crackers and spring rolls; noodle dishes; sweet and sour dishes, or anything in batter.

Egypt/Middle East

Choose: crudités and dips, such as hummous or baba ghanoush; grilled meats and fish, such as kebabs or shashlik; salads; stuffed vegetables and vine leaves; tagines; rice dishes.

Refuse: couscous and flat breads; deep-fried falafel and fatayer; tabbouleh; pastries; Turkish delight.

France

Choose: French onion soup (without the bread on top) or bouillabaisse fish soup; a seafood platter; omelettes; beef bourguignon; cassoulet; steak, chicken and fish dishes with salads.

Refuse: bread and cow's cheeses; croissants; cream sauces; Lyonnaise potatoes (full of cream); pastry; crêpes; patisserie.

Greece/Cyprus

Choose: Greek salad, dips with chopped vegetable crudités; olives; kebabs; lamb kleftiko; dolmades (vine leaves stuffed with rice); stifado (a casserole with beef or game); souvlaki (meat and vegetables on skewers); all kinds of freshly grilled fish and seafood.

Refuse: pitta bread; deep-fried pastries such as spanakopita; moussaka; sweets.

India

Choose: tandoori dishes with salad; raitas; lentil dishes such as dahl; chickpea and bean curries; vegetable curries and rice dishes; tomato-based or dry meat, chicken and fish curries.

Refuse: deep-fried samosas, bhajis and pakora; naan bread and chapattis, popadoms; kormas, which have a creamy sauce, and Keralan curries, which tend to be cooked in high-calorie coconut milk sauces; gulab jamun (a sweet dessert).

Italy

Choose: antipasti, such as figs with Parma ham, or chargrilled artichokes; salads; stews, such as chicken cacciatore; grilled meat, fish and chicken with vegetables; risotto (although it's always best to check with the waiter as they can often be very creamy and cheesey).

Refuse: pizza; pasta; bread and polenta; ice cream (except as a very occasional treat); cappuccino.

Japan

Choose: miso soup; sushi, sashimi and nori rolls; seaweed salad; teppanyaki dishes (fish or meat with vegetables); tofu dishes; rice and rice noodles.

Refuse: tempura dishes (deep-fried in batter); teriyaki sauce (very sweet).

Mexico/Caribbean

Choose: guacamole and salsa; salads; all kinds of fish and seafood; chicken and meat; chilli con carne with rice; refried beans; spicy chicken wings; tacos made from corn (check with the waiter that they are wheat-free).

Refuse: tortillas and nachos.

Spain

Choose: gazpacho; paella; omelettes; seafood and chicken stews; fabada asturiana (a bean stew); freshly grilled fish and seafood.

Refuse: calamari (or anything deep-fried in batter); bread; fideuà (noodles); pastries and flans.

Thailand

Choose: tom yam soup; salads; stir-fried fish, chicken and meat dishes with herbs and spices; rice and rice noodles (phat); steamed fish and seafood dishes.

Refuse: spring rolls; red and green curries (that are cooked in high-fat coconut milk sauces); wheat noodles (khao) ;anything deep-fried.

Turkey

Choose: kebabs and koftas; imam bayildi (stuffed aubergine); all kinds of stuffed vegetables; salads and pilaf rice dishes; meat stews with fruit.

Refuse: bread and pastries; bulgar wheat.

United States

Choose: any items from self-service salad bars that aren't deep-fried or drowned in mayonnaise; baked potatoes instead of chips; local specialities such as lobster in New England or jambalaya in New Orleans; grilled steaks (without the creamy sauce on top).

Refuse: the bun that comes with the burger or hot dog; pizza; pecan pie (or any kind of pie for that matter).

Staying active on holiday

You could lie on a sun lounger for two weeks and only move when it's time for another feed, but you would soon feel your muscle tone melting away and new reserves of lard forming beneath you. Alternatively, you could incorporate some physical activity into your holiday in a way that means you keep up the positive progress you've made – and it could help to make your trip more fun as well. It's a no-brainer, if you ask us.

Here are some ways of staying trim and toned and having fun at the same time.

In the pool

- Walk around the shallow end making your legs work against the resistance of the water.
- Buy a pair of bats and a little ball and get someone to play with you. Hit the ball high so you both have to jump to reach it.
- Some pools have a net so you can play water volleyball, or sets of goals so you can play water polo.
- Your resort may offer aquafit or aquarobics classes in the pool – or you could do your own session with your friends using the exercises on page 123.
- Alternatively, just swim some fast, competitive lengths up and down the pool every day.

In the sea

- Find out about the watersports available and consider trying waterskiing, surfing, windsurfing, kayaking, body boarding – or taking out a pedalo.
- If there are big waves on your beach, stand and jump or dive through them, letting them pummel your flesh.
- Play ball games in the water – simple throwing and catching requires a lot more effort in waves than in the pool.
- Walk in hip-high water for the length of the beach.
- Swim the length of the beach – after checking that it is safe to do so.

On the sand

- Walking and running are much more effective calorie burners on sand, and really good for toning your legs and butt as well. Why not get up early and have a run along the shore before breakfast every day?
- Practise cartwheels and handstands on the sand. Try to get back the proficiency you had in youth.
- Join in that game of beach volleyball. It's tough on the calves and thighs, but it's how the girls in Rio de Janeiro tone their fabulous derrières to perfection.
- Fling a frisbee.
- Even a game of boules will get you off your butt and moving around.

Around the resort

- Hire a bike and explore the area on two wheels.
- Find out about trekking and horse-riding options.
- Climb a mountain or volcano.
- Try white-water rafting.
- Dance the night away in a local club.

If you're simply too embarrassed to exercise in public, have a mini aerobic workout in your hotel room using the routine described on pages 132–135.

Wherever you are, there are bound to be some fun options for keeping the muscle tone you worked so hard to achieve. The more you do, the fitter you'll look, the better you'll feel. And you'll also be able to burn off any excess calories you might find yourself taking in as you sample the local delicacies.

Going for the burn

There is one benefit to being overweight – just one – and that is that you burn more calories than your skinny friends when doing exactly the same thing. Even lying on a sun lounger flicking through the pages of a magazine, you are using more energy than the slim friend next to you, because your body has more tissues to look after. Women tend to burn fewer calories than men of the same weight because they usually have less muscle. And sadly we all burn fewer calories as we get older.

When working out roughly how many calories a person burns from a particular exercise or activity, it's important to take their body weight into consideration. The chart below looks at people who are 77 kg (12 stone), 102 kg (16 stone) and 127 kg (20 stone). Choose the one that is closest to your weight to get an idea what you would have to do.

To burn off a typical full English breakfast (715 kcal):
- A 77-kg (12-stone) person would have to climb stairs for 1 hour 34 minutes.
- A 102-kg (16-stone) person would have to climb stairs for 1 hour 10 minutes.
- A 127-kg (20-stone) person would have to climb stairs for 56 minutes.

To burn off a single scoop of chocolate ice cream in a cone (283 kcal):
- A 77-kg (12-stone) person would have to skip for 20 minutes.
- A 102-kg (16-stone) person would have to skip for 15 minutes.
- A 127-kg (20-stone) person would have to skip for 12 minutes.

To burn off a four-cheese pizza (636 kcal):
- A 77-kg (12-stone) person would have to run for 40 minutes.
- A 102-kg (16-stone) person would have to run for 30 minutes.
- A 127-kg (20-stone) person would have to run for 24 minutes.

To burn off a pina colada (280 kcal):
- A 77-kg (12-stone) person would have to waterski for 37 minutes.
- A 102-kg (16-stone) person would have to waterski for 28 minutes.
- A 127-kg (20-stone) person would have to waterski for 22 minutes.

To burn off a portion of fish and chips (465 kcal):
- A 77-kg (12-stone) person would have to swim for 59 minutes.
- A 102-kg (16-stone) person would have to swim for 46 minutes.
  A 127-kg (20-stone) person would have to swim for 37 minutes.

To burn off a portion of lasagne (669 kcal):
- A 77-kg (12-stone) person would have to play volleyball for
  1 hour 45 minutes.
- A 102-kg (16-stone) person would have to play volleyball for
  1 hour 19 minutes.
- A 127-kg (20-stone) person would have to play volleyball for
  1 hour 3 minutes.

To burn off a large slice of Black Forest Gâteau (840 kcal):
- A 77-kg (12-stone) person would have to cycle for 1 hour 50 minutes.
- A 102-kg (16-stone) person would have to cycle for 1 hour
  22 minutes.
- A 127-kg (20-stone) person would have to cycle for 1 hour 6 minutes.

If you slip up on holiday and don't want to return to some scarily big numbers on the bathroom scales, consider introducing your own calorie-burn system. The morning after a heavy night, slip out of bed and decide how you can do some serious burning to get you back to where you were before. Choose an efficient method such as running, skipping or fast cycling rather than simply trying to swim yourself slim with a few sedate lengths of the pool.

After all you've been through, it would be a shame to let one night of excess set you back on the road to being a lardy ass again. If you completed the Beach Body Blitz, you are a strong, determined person with the ability to get your weight and your health under control long term. Now is your chance to prove it!

CHAPTER SIX

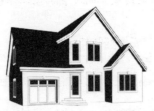

Back home again

It's decision time. As you unpack your suitcase and shake the sand out of your beach towel, take a moment to reflect on whether you would prefer to let your figure get flabby again, safe in the knowledge that you can always do a Beach Body Blitz before the next holiday – or if you would like to start being a fit, healthy person from now on.

It's a classic case of double cheeseburger versus healthy arteries, chocolate chip cookies versus slender thighs, and five pints of bitter versus toned abdominals. Which way do you want to go?

OK, so far we've held off on the lectures about what excess weight does to your health. But here are a few facts:

- If you are obese you are twice as likely to have high blood pressure as someone of a healthy weight.
- Being overweight makes you more likely to die of heart disease or stroke without experiencing any warning signs beforehand. You could just drop dead.

- Overweight people are twice as likely to develop type 2 diabetes.
- Women who have gained more than 9 kg (20 lb) since the age of eighteen are twice as likely to get breast cancer.
- Overweight men are at significantly greater risk of cancers of the colon, rectum and prostate.
- You are much more likely to get osteoarthritis in your hips, knees and lower back if you are carrying excess weight.
- The risk of getting gallstones is three times higher if you are obese.

We could go on – but basically, you are likely to die younger than someone who is a healthy weight. Your lifestyle is chopping years off your life expectancy. Are you happy about that? Or do you want to do something about it?

The good news is that losing as little as 10 percent of your body weight can dramatically reduce the risks, and getting down to a healthy BMI score (see page 208) could well put you back on a level playing field with your slimmer friends.

Wouldn't you like to turn back the clock to a time before you got overweight? Why not do it now, when you've already got a head start?

If horror statistics about health risks don't do it for you, how about plain vanity? You looked good in beachwear but maybe you could still look better in your everyday clothes. Wouldn't you like to wear a pair of jeans without a roll of flesh curving over the top? Girls, think of all those fabulous figure-hugging party dresses you never even try on because you don't want to look like a squashed blancmange oozing over the edges of the tub. Guys, if you currently wear baggy shirts to camouflage the moobs, think how great it will be to choose slimline, tailored ones again.

You've come back from your beach holiday rested and relaxed, with renewed energy and enthusiasm for life. All you need to do now is direct a little bit of that energy into creating some healthy habits that will fit into your normal lifestyle and become second nature. It's not that hard. Slim people do it as a matter of course – and you can too.

What is your ideal weight range?

Most doctors still use body mass index as a measure of whether you are a healthy weight for your height. It's not a perfect system because, for example, if you are heavily muscled you may creep into an overweight category, but it's a useful general guide.

To calculate your body mass index, you need to know your weight in kilograms (or stones) and your height in metres (or feet), then check the chart on page 208 to see where you fall on the scale:

- **Over 40 means you are severely obese.**
- **Between 30 and 40 is obese.**
- **Between 25 and 30 is overweight.**
- **Between 19 and 25 is the healthy weight range.**
- **Between 15 and 19 means you are underweight.**
- **A score of less than 15 means you are emaciated.**

If you scored over 40 or under 15 you should seek medical advice straight away because your health is at risk.

If your BMI is over 30, you should do all you can to get it back down to a healthier range. There's advice on how to do it and how long it should take in the following pages. Why not make use of the advice on The Biggest Loser Club website (www.biggestloserclub.co.uk)?

If your BMI is between 25 and 30, use the chart on page 208 to find out what weight you would need to get down to for a healthy BMI score. How much weight would you have to lose? Once again, see page 209 for advice on how long it should take to get there.

If your BMI is under 19, you need to make sure you are eating three meals a day and covering all the food groups and are taking in a reasonable amount of calories per day. It may be that you are naturally rake-like but keep an eye on your weight and don't let it drop too low.

And, if your BMI is between 19 and 25, pat yourself on the back. All you need to do is ensure you stay there by making sensible eating and exercise a part of your everyday lifestyle (see pages 217–218).

BMI chart

In the example given, a person with a height of 5'7" and weighing 13 stone can be seen to be overweight.

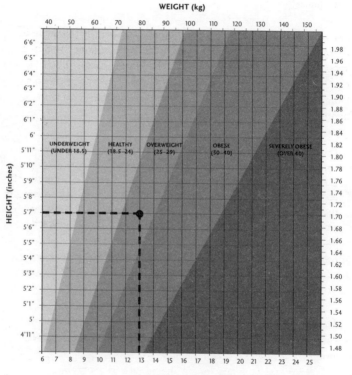

More weight to lose?

Is your BMI sky-high? Still got several stone to lose? The main thing is not to set yourself unrealistic goals then beat yourself up when you don't meet them. Slow and steady is the way to go if you want to keep that weight off for good, and it can help if you break your goal down into chunks.

Say you currently weigh 127 kg (20 stone) and want to get down to 77 kg (12 stone). You have 50 kg (8 stone) to lose, which sounds an impossibly huge amount. A realistic rate of weight loss is 0.5–1 kg (1–2 pounds) a week, so it could take you two years to reach your target, and it's difficult to keep your motivation over such a long period. Try this instead.

- GOAL NO. 1 – lose 10 percent of your body weight, i.e. 12 kg (2 stone), within 6 months. This is a manageable amount. In fact, you will probably reach this target much sooner if you follow the eating and exercise advice on pages 211–214. So within 6 months of your starting date, you should weigh 115 kg (18 stone). When you get there, have a rest for a week. Don't go back to eating the massive amounts of food that made you the size you are, but let yourself have a few more 'treats' – just for a week.
- GOAL NO. 2 – lose the next 13 kg (2 stone) in the same amount of time that it took you to achieve Goal No. 1. Then you'll be down to 102 kg (16 stone). Again, take a week off.
- GOAL NO. 3 – get to 89 kg (14 stone) in the same time again. Take a week off.
- GOAL NO. 4 – reach your target weight. Switch to a maintenance level of eating and exercise (see pages 217–218).

Each time you start a new goal, recalculate the daily calorie intake you are aiming at, because it will decrease as you get lighter and your body doesn't need so many calories to perform its basic functions.

Goal no. 1 should be to lose no more than 10 percent of your current weight, at a rate of 0.5–1 kg (1–2 pounds) a week. Decide on your start date and get going!

Keeping a weight-loss diary

If you have space in your Beach Body Blitz notebook, you can continue the story of your weight-loss journey in there. Otherwise, buy a new notebook and paste in some pictures from the holiday, showing you in swimwear as you are now. Jot down your measurements and weight, and write your Weight Loss Goal No. 1 in big letters.

Each day, write down everything you eat and drink (apart from water and sugar- and milk-free coffee and tea). This is important because it's all too easy to forget about the odd biscuit here and there, or the leftover fish finger you polished off before washing up the kids' dinner plates, but they all have calorie consequences. If the weight isn't dropping off as quickly as you'd like, the reason will be in these pages. Quite simply, you must still be eating too much.

You should also jot down each exercise session you take, whether fat-burning or resistance exercise, to make sure you achieve the total number of sessions you are aiming at each week (see page 215).

Don't weigh yourself every day. Weight loss can fluctuate according to factors such as water retention, menstruation (for women), and normal hormonal action for both sexes. Step on the scales once a week, first thing in the morning, without clothes on, and jot down the figures in your notebook. If the numbers haven't dropped for two weeks in a row, check back through your food diary to see where you have been over-indulging. Use a calorie counter to figure out where you're going wrong (see page 212).

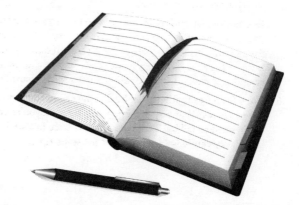

Healthy eating for weight loss

To lose weight, you need to burn more calories through exercise than you take in through food. That's the bottom line. But how can you judge how much to eat, so that you lose weight yet still get all the nutrients your body needs? Either you will have to follow a set diet such as *The Biggest Loser: Permanent Weight Loss Plan*, or you will have to learn the basics about food and nutrition yourself.

Here are some golden rules to help you.

1   Eat regular meals. Don't let more than 4 hours go by without eating a meal or a snack or you could find that hunger and low blood sugar propel you towards high-calorie food choices.

2   Never skip breakfast. It kick-starts your metabolism for the day. Opt for a high-fibre cereal with dried fruit and skimmed milk, some fresh fruit and yogurt, or a poached egg with spinach on wholemeal toast.

3   Eat balanced meals. At lunch and dinner, cover half your plate with vegetables or salad, a quarter with a lean source of protein (fish, chicken, tofu, eggs, or occasional portions of lean red meat), and a quarter with a healthy carbohydrate (brown rice, wholemeal bread, couscous). If your weight loss isn't as fast as it should be, cut starchy carbs with your evening meal, replacing them with extra vegetables instead.

4   Write down everything you eat in your weight-loss notebook (see page 18). If you slip up and guzzle a chocolate biscuit, try to understand why. Were you experiencing a mid-afternoon blood sugar dip? Were you bored? Understanding should help you to avoid temptation in future.

5   Choose low-fat options whenever you can. Low-fat milk, cheese and yogurt are lower in calories too. Cut the visible fat off meat and take the skin off chicken or turkey. Use a spray of olive oil for cooking rather than a glug of a less healthy oil. Spread your bread with a scraping of olive-oil spread rather than a thick layer of butter.

6   Cook from fresh rather than buying packaged ready meals and jarred sauces. That way you know exactly what you're consuming. If you need to fall back on instant foods once in a while, read the labels very carefully (see page 214 for some tips).

7   Plan meals ahead of time and organize your shopping so that
    you   always have plenty of nutritious food in the house. Don't go
    shopping on an empty stomach or it can lead you to the wrong
    aisles in the supermarket.

8   Dump the worst kinds of sugary, salty, fatty junk food. Just don't
    give them house room. Be particularly strict about avoiding the
    types of food that made you fat in the first place. Go on – you know
    exactly what they are!

9   Having said that, you won't be able to stick to your diet if it's denial
    all the way so allow yourself a 100-calorie treat per day. This could
    be a small glass (125ml/4 fl oz) of wine, a half pint (300 ml/½ pint)
    of beer, two squares (25 g/1 oz) of chocolate, or a small (50 g/
    2 oz) portion of ice cream.

10 Keep active. As well as your regular exercise sessions (see page 215),
    take every opportunity you can to burn calories during the day and
    avoid long periods of sitting in front of a computer or the TV. Walk
    around while you're on the phone instead of curling up in an
    armchair. Climb every staircase. Play football with the kids.

Planning your meals

There are various ways to calculate how many calories you should be
taking in per day, but we are going to make it simple. The following
calculation assumes that you are getting three weekly sessions of fat-
burning exercise and at least 60 minutes of moderate physical activity
per day, through walking, housework, or resistance exercise sessions.

• For women: multiply your weight in kilos by 33. This gives the number
  of calories you need to maintain the same weight. To lose weight at
  a rate of 0.5 kg (1 pound) per week, subtract 500 from this, and
  you've got your target daily intake. So for example, if you are a
  woman weighing 70 kg (11 stone), your daily intake should be
  (70 x 33) – 500 = 1,810 kcals.
• For men: multiply your weight in kilos by 37. This gives the number
  of calories you need to maintain the same weight. To lose weight at
  a rate of 0.5kg (1 pound) per week, subtract 500 from this, and
  you've got your target daily intake. If you are a man weighing 100 kg
  (16 stone), your daily intake should be (100 x 37) – 500 = 3,200 kcals.

You can go a bit lower than this if you want (so long as you are getting
enough nutrients) but never go below 1,500 kcal a day for women
and 1,750 kcal for men except under medical supervision.

Spread your calorie intake throughout the day. Here's how you might spread a daily intake of 2,000 kcal.

Breakfast of 400 kcal
Mid-morning snack of 150 kcal
Lunch of up to 600 kcal
Mid-afternoon snack of 150 kcal
Dinner of up to 600 kcal
'Treat' of 100 kcal

Adjust this to suit your lifestyle and the times of day when you tend to feel hungriest. You may even find there are days when you don't manage to consume your full calorie allowance. Give yourself a big fat tick in your notebook when you come in under budget, so to speak.

Once you become calorie aware, you won't need to count every last carrot stick (one medium carrot has 35 kcal, by the way). But until then, it is worth investing in a handbag-sized calorie counter or getting a calorie-counting app on your phone. Tot up your calorie totals in your food diary to check that you are keeping within the limits. It will soon be second nature to size up that extra slice of buttered toast and ask yourself whether you can afford another 170 or so kcal.

Avoid 'empty' calories. Try to make sure that everything you eat contains some kind of nutrient that your body needs.

The main thing is to learn which foods are healthy and low in calories, and opt for them rather than foods that are high in calories but with no nutritional value whatsoever. You may find that, without even trying, you have revised your whole approach to food – from changing your shopping habits to enjoying preparing and cooking fresh food that you take pleasure in eating and sharing with family and friends. Everyone benefits, and not only for those few weeks before you jet off to the sun, but all year round.

READING FOOD LABELS

Even with the new traffic lights system introduced by supermarkets and manufacturers, food labels can be misleading. Read the small print carefully to find out whether the calorie count they are giving is per 100 g (3½ oz) of the food or per 'portion'. If it's per portion, how big is a portion? Is it half the pack? Or one slice? If it's per 100 g (3½ oz), is it clear how much of the food constitutes 100 g (3½ oz)? Sometimes you have to become a food detective to find out.

Some foods may get a red 'high calorie' traffic light, but still be fine to eat in moderation. Nuts, for example, contain a lot of fat, so they are a fattening food, but their healthy nutrients mean it's still worth having two or three in your breakfast cereal.

Be aware that ingredients on packaged food are listed in order of the quantity of them the product contains. This helps you to avoid sausages if the first item on the list isn't meat, or yogurts that have more sugar than fruit!

Nutritional Facts

Serving Size 1 cookie (16g)
Serving Per Customer 27

Amount Per Serving	
Calories 80	Calories from fat 30

% Daily Value*	
Total Fat 3.5g	5%
Saturated Fat 1.5g	8%
Trans Fat 0.5g	
Cholestorol 0mg	0%
Sodium 40mg	2%
Total Carbohydrate 11g	4%
Dietry Fibre 0g	0%
Sugar 5g	
Protein Less than 1g	

Vitamin A 0%	•	Vitamin C 0%
Calcium 0%	•	Iron 4%

Percent Daily Values are based on a 2000 calorie diet. You Daily Values may be higher or lower depending on your calorie needs.

Serving size
Note that the serving size here is just one cookie.

Calories
Here the calories per serving are given, rather than per 100 g (3½ oz).

% daily value
This tells you what percentage of the maximum recommended amount is included in a portion of the product. If you are trying to lose weight, you should, of course, be consuming less fat and fewer calories than this recommended value.

***Trans* fat**
It's best to avoid any product that contains these.

Sodium
This is salt. Keep your intake as low as you can.

Exercise for weight loss

In all long-term studies of people who have lost significant amounts of weight, it's the ones who adopted exercise as part of their lifestyle who kept the weight off. Exercise keeps your metabolism burning plenty of calories so you get away with the odd slip-up food-wise. And while you are in a weight-loss programme, a varied, energetic exercise schedule can double the rate at which you shed the flab.

In a longer-term programme, you don't need to make the 2½-hours-a-day commitment that you did during the Beach Body Blitz. All you need to do is 3 hour-long sessions a week of fat-burning and resistance exercise, and make sure you are active for at least an hour every single day. This could mean walking to the shops, vacuuming the stairs, or maybe doing some gardening. If there's a day when you are stuck at your desk most of the time, do the Resistance Workout or an exercise DVD at home in the evening.

As before, choose the aerobic, fat-burning exercise you like – whatever is handy and fits in with your lifestyle. For the resistance exercise sessions, follow the plan on pages 136–185 or ask the trainer at your gym to work out a routine for you. Don't forget to do warm-ups and cool-downs before and after every aerobic session.

Pick the time of day that suits you to exercise. It could be first thing in the morning, at lunchtime, or after work in the evening. If you're lucky enough to be self-employed you can go out during the quietest times of day when everyone else is in the office.

Just make sure you get in those three sessions a week come rain or shine, and you'll be dramatically increasing your rate of weight loss as well as making yourself healthier all round.

Your Beach Body Blitz will have given you a head start and got you used to an active lifestyle and sensible eating choices. Now you know you can make a real difference to your body without starving and giving up normal life, you should be able to get rid of those remaining kilos (pounds) without too much of a struggle.

Weight loss do's

- Eat regular, balanced meals and snacks.

- Plan your meals, and always keep a stock of healthy, nutritious foods in your kitchen.

- If you are eating out, choose plain, good-quality grilled fish, chicken and meat dishes rather than concoctions with heavy, creamy sauces.

- If you are unsure about the calorie content of a food, look it up in a calorie counter. As a general rule, sweet and fatty foods will be the high-calorie ones but there are exceptions.

- Stick roughly to the portion sizes given in the recipes in this book. Even if you are eating only healthy foods, you will still put on weight if you eat too much of them.

- Do continue to avoid wheat, cow's milk and cheese, booze, red meat or sugar if you felt better after excluding them on the Beach Body Blitz, or at least cut down significantly.

- Do vary your exercise programme, trying different sports or activities to keep it interesting.

- Keep congratulating yourself for every kilo (pound) lost. Remember that you have just reduced your risk of serious illness and premature death by a fraction, as well as made yourself look better.

Weight loss don'ts

- Don't skip meals, because the blood sugar dip will make you crave the wrong kinds of foods.

- Don't exclude whole food groups, such as carbs, because this will have all kinds of negative effects on your health before long.

- Don't skip exercise sessions. Once you begin, it's a slippery slope and you'll find yourself making excuses more and more often. These three sessions a week should be an integral part of your life now, like brushing your teeth and doing the laundry. They are just something you have to do to stay healthy.

- Don't deny yourself treats. That one treat a day is psychologically very important.

- Don't weigh yourself obsessively; once a week is enough.

- Don't lose heart if your weight loss appears to stall at any stage. Check your food intake in your notebook and if it is all in order, just carry on and your weight will begin to drop again before long.

- Don't repeat the Beach Body Blitz fortnight more than once every six months.

Maintaining your healthy weight for life

We all have a natural healthy weight, the weight our bodies want us to be, and when we reach that we will maintain it without too much effort. There's no point in struggling to fit into tiny sizes if your frame is simply too large. You just won't make it without starving yourself to the point of malnutrition.

You may reach a weight that is healthy on the BMI scale but feel you still want to get rid of some flabby bits. In this case, exercise is the way to go. Recalculate your daily calorie intake for your new weight and keep doing your three exercise sessions a week, performing extra repetitions of the resistance exercises that target the area you're unhappy with. Some types of fat, such as post-pregnancy belly fat, can take ages to shift but if you persevere you will see improvements.

When you reach your target weight, don't think you can now reintroduce all the junk foods that made you overweight in the first place unless you want to be right back at square one.

If you continue to eat healthily, with just the odd indulgence, and keep exercising regularly, maintaining a healthy weight should happen naturally.

At first you might want to work out the number of calories you should be consuming per day for your new weight, and keep an eye on your intake, but soon it will become instinctive. In the old days, when you looked at a chocolate éclair, you either thought, 'That looks delicious; I'm going to treat myself,' or 'That would be lovely but I won't have it because I don't want to break my diet.' The new you will look at that same éclair and think 'It's a big old chunk of animal fat, sugar and processed white flour with absolutely no nutritional value and containing 297 kcals.' You may remember that it was momentarily satisfying to eat, but you know you would have a blood sugar dip shortly afterwards and decide it's not worth using up such a high percentage of your daily calorie intake on one unhealthy item. This is how slim people think.

Of course, no one's perfect. There may be periods when you slip up and put on a bit of weight again. Christmas is a notorious danger zone. The sooner you stop the backwards slide and get back to eating well, the easier it will be to return to your healthy weight. After a bit of backsliding, it's a good idea to dig out your trusty weight loss notebook and keep track of what you eat and how much you exercise. Putting it down in black and white will focus your efforts.

The key thing is to decide that this newly slim body is the one that you want to take with you for the rest of your life. The skin may wrinkle over the decades but by keeping to a healthy weight, you are statistically likely to have a much easier time of it healthwise as you get older, and you are also likely to live longer. You'll look good in your clothes and have more energy to enjoy yourself with friends and family.

And when booking your next beach holiday, you won't have a moment's hesitation. You'll be able to try different styles of swimwear and choose the ones you like rather than the ones that camouflage your excess. When you step out onto the sand, people will glance up from their sun lounger and think 'There's someone who looks after themselves.' Wouldn't that be nice?

Remember: by next year's beach holiday you will have the body you deserve.

Index

Stockists

For wheat-free bread and rolls:
www.wheatanddairyfree.com
www.dietaryspecials.co.uk
www.goodness.co.uk
www.goodnessdirect.co.uk

For advice on running, and buying running shoes:
www.runnersworld.co.uk
www.momentumsports.co.uk

For advice on cycling, and buying a bike:
www.whycycle.co.uk
http://bicycling.about.com/od/howtoride/a/right_bike.htm

To buy skipping ropes:
www.skip-hop.co.uk

To buy rollerblades:
www.rollerblade.com

To buy trampolines:
www.trampolinesonline.co.uk

To buy hula hoops:
www.hoopswhirled.com/hoop_shop.shtml

For information about Wii Fit:
http://wiifit.com

To buy hand-held weights, resistance bands and steps:
www.escapefitness.com
www.weightlossresources.co.uk/shop
www.resistancebands.org.uk

Picture credits

Cover front, Jon Feingersh/Getty Images; back, Stockbrokerxtra Images/Photolibrary; background, Walter Quirtmair/Fotolia.com

Jaz Bahra 15 below, 57 left, 60 left, 60 right, 64 left, 69 left, 75 bottom, 90 centre above, 90 centre, 90 centre below, 90 right, 93, 96, 98, 103, 187, 188 above, 205.

Fotolia/Albachiaraa 30; /allison 14–15 (except 15 below), 57 right, 60 centre below, 75 above right; /Oleg Averin 64 centre above, 64 centre below, 64 right, 69 centre, 75 above left; /Bojanovic78 122; /Slobodan Djajic 108; /Anastasija Dracova 22; /draganm 195; /drizzd 10; /dvarg 111; /Fica 38; /Guilu 90 above left, 90 centre right; /Adrian Hillman 130–1; /hippo 138, 146; /JungleOutThere 188–9 (except 188 above); /Kamaga 196; /Mannaggia 24; /Anna Marinova 43 centre, 60 centre above, 79 above centre; /Anton Novikov 119; /Irina Onufrieva 210; /patrimonio designs 43 right, 79 left; /Svetlana Romanova 69 right, 79 right; /SahinMurat 166; /Massimo Saivezzo 160, 174; /Santi 112 (reused throughout), 128; /Snaptitude 154; /Wichittra Srisunon 13, 186; /Vadym Tynenko 43 left; /Luisa Venturoli 6.

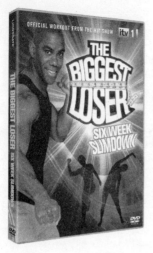

The perfect exercise routines to optimize your weight loss!

You've seen the incredible weight loss achieved on ITV1's hit show, 'The Biggest Loser'. Now, just like the contestants, you too can shed the pounds and experience stunning weight loss right from your living room! Join The Biggest Loser training professional, Richard Callender, as he takes on the role of your personal trainer in 'The Biggest Loser: Six Week Slimdown'.

AVAILABLE NOW ON DVD!

Biggest Loser Meal Replacements

Become a weight-loss winner with The Biggest Loser today! It's easy – simply replace two meals a day with a shake, soup or bar. You can then enjoy healthy, satisfying snacks in between meals and a delicious balanced meal for dinner.

Each Biggest Loser 'meal' is specially formulated to be low in calories and rich in nutrients and vitamins, so you feel satisfied and get the nutritional balance you need.

The Biggest Loser Meal Replacements are:

- High in protein – to help maintain muscle mass and keep your metabolism revving.

- Low GI – our shakes and soups help you feel fuller for longer.

- Calorie controlled – to help you achieve the energy balance that is required for weight management.

- Delicious and easy – to prepare our shakes and soups, just add water!

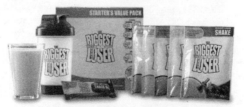

For more information and recipe ideas, please visit **www.biggestloserclub.co.uk**